# *Performance* MASSAGE

## Robert K. King
AMTA Certified Massage Therapist

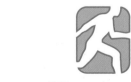

**Human Kinetics Publishers**

**Library of Congress Cataloging-in Publication Data**

King, Robert K., 1948-
    Performance massage / Robert K. King
      p.  cm.
    Includes bibliographical references (p. ).
    ISBN 0-87322-395-0
    1. Massage.  2. Sports.  3. Athletes.  I. Title
  RM721.K36  1992
  615.8'22--dc20

92- 12303
CIP

ISBN: 0-87322-395-0

Developmental Editor: Holly Gilly
Managing Editor: Marni Basic
Assistant Editors: Laura Bofinger, Moyra Knight, & Julie Swadener
Copyeditor: Wendy Nelson
Proofreader: Karin Leszcyznski
Indexer: Theresa J. Schaefer
Production Director: Ernie Noa
Typesetter and Text Layout: Kathleen Boudreau-Fuoss
Text Design: Keith Blomberg
Cover Design: Jack Davis
Cover and Interior Photos: Wilmer Zehr
Interior Art: Doug Burnett
Models: Mike Berger, Dawn Campbell, Lydia Chin, and Jason Hood
Printer: Sung in America

Human Kinetics books are available at special discounts for bulk purchase for sales promotions, premiums, fund-raising, or educational use. Special editions or book excerpts can also be created to specification. For details, contact the Special Sales Manager at Human Kinetics.

Printed in Korea

10  9  8  7  6  5  4  3  2  1

**Human Kinetics Publishers**
Box 5076, Champaign, IL 61825-5076
1-800-747-4457

*Canada Office:*
Human Kinetics Publishers, Inc.
P.O. Box 2503, Windsor, ON
  N8Y 4S2
1-800-465-7301 (in Canada only)

*Europe Office:*
Human Kinetics Publishers (Europe) Ltd.
P.O. Box IW14
Leeds LS16 6TR
England    0532-781708

*Australia Office:*
Human Kinetics Publishers
P.O. Box 80
Kingswood 5062
South Australia    374-0433

# Contents

# Foreword

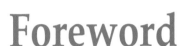began to use massage in 1980 when I was preparing for the Boston Marathon, and I've been hooked on it ever since. I injured myself during training in 1988 and used massage as part of my rehabilitation. I'm convinced that it helped speed my recovery. As I've grown older and begun competing in Masters events, I find regular massage more and more important for preventing injuries.

As a marathon runner, I find that a massage 2 to 3 days before a competition helps me warm up better, and massage after a run is a wonderful way to flush out and rejuvenate my tired muscles. My favorite time for massage, though, is neither just before nor after training, but during my regular weekly session. The time I spend on the massage table is relaxing but energizing.

Even if I weren't an athlete who trains regularly, I would still use massage to keep my muscles in shape for any kind of physical activity. It's a gift I give myself for being committed to a healthy lifestyle.

I think it's great that now there's a book that teaches people how to do the kind of massage that will help them take care of their muscles. I hope you'll take the time to learn the techniques in *Performance Massage* and use them as a regular part of your workout program or activity schedule. Your body will thank you!

Bill Rodgers
  4-time winner of the Boston Marathon and New York Marathon

# Preface

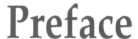hat do Ringo Star, Jackie Joyner-Kersee, Greg LeMond, Bob Hope, Boomer Esiason, George Bush, Chuck Norris, Joan Benoit Samuelson and Rudolf Nureyev have in common?

They all utilize massage therapy to enhance their wellness, athletic, physical fitness, or artistic performance programs.

Public acceptance of massage therapy, at least in the United States, has been slow in arriving. Some people still snicker or raise their eyebrows when massage therapists describe their occupation. Massage has been variously associated with run-down bathhouses, New Age cults, "massage parlors," or some mysterious laying on of hands. Many of us have been ignorant of the therapeutic benefits of touch more than anything else.

Fortunately, this situation is changing. Massage therapy is an emerging profession, and the number of practitioners, schools, and recipients is steadily increasing.

In 1985, the leading massage therapy organization, the American Massage Therapy Association (AMTA), established a sports massage certification program and national team following the successful volunteer massage effort at the 1984 Olympiad in Los Angeles. AMTA's program underscores sports massage as a specialized field featuring therapeutic approaches specific to the stress, strain, and overuse syndromes common to activity.

The AMTA initiative introduced massage to the contemporary generation of athletes and fitness enthusiasts. Therapeutic massage is now offered at the Olympic Games, the Pan American Games, the Goodwill Games, and major marathons, triathlons, and sporting events.

The fitness community's acceptance of professional massage was graphically illustrated to me at the conclusion of the 1985 Chicago Marathon. As one of the AMTA volunteer team, I was performing cool-down massage in the elite runners' tent. Joan Benoit Samuelson, who had astounded the sporting community the previous year by winning the Olympic Marathon in record time a few weeks after knee surgery, easily won the women's division in Chicago's grueling 26-mile run. After crossing the finish line, Joan made her way to the massage tent, and we began performing the very techniques you'll be learning in this book. Her commitment to massage therapy was underscored by her keeping the media, the race directors, and her husband all waiting while she received massage on her exhausted leg and back muscles. As a massage practitioner, I began to feel our time had come.

Nurturing, knowledgeable touch is now validated by research and clinical studies as a powerful therapeutic agent. More importantly, it is available to all of us.

My own interest in performance massage stems from the muscle strains, sprains, injuries, and surgeries that have plagued my athletic career. As a former boxer, runner, competitive weight lifter, and sport participant I experienced more than my share of downtime. I began searching for ways to eradicate the lingering effects of muscle injuries and for preventive measures as well.

Over the past 20 years I have worked with world class athletes, thousands of weekend warriors, and many dancers in a number of different settings. What I have found is that the impact of repetitive movements and muscle strain takes a cumulative toll on the body's connective tissues.

Fitness buffs, athletes, and performing artists interested in peak performance need massage therapy techniques that enhance movement, flexibility, and optimal muscle functioning. What I have assembled in *Performance Massage* is a specialized approach to lengthening, stretching, and unwinding these physical distortions and restrictions encountered by active people.

Movement—whether the whirling heave of the shot-putter, the intricate shoulder mechanics of a 95-mph fastball, the graceful spin of a pirouette, or the repetitive motion of an aerobic dance routine—is the essence of activity. I have designed an approach that uses movement as a key component of massage therapy. I synthesize muscle stretching movements with skillful hands-on therapeutics, creating a dynamic relationship between physical function and structure.

*Performance Massage* is written for all physically active people, including those who pursue a sport or dance regularly. My intent is to provide you with fundamental touch skills and techniques that enhance performance, reduce injuries, and complement high-level wellness. Through Performance Massage, you can enhance athletic longevity, increase overall performance, and reduce the muscular soreness and congestion that frequently inhibit free and graceful range of motion.

I believe that anyone can perform a basic, effective hands-on massage session by following certain guidelines, precautions, and directions. Touching skills are inherent in all of us, and appropriate techniques and stretches can be learned by anyone willing to practice the techniques in this book.

The Performance Massage sequence is presented in a system that is user-friendly. In other words, it feels great! It taps into our inherent capacity of touch and targets the athlete in all of us who wants to perform more effectively at an optimal level.

Applying the techniques of this book is one of many steps you can take as part of a lifetime commitment to fitness, physical activity, and sport participation. I have experienced excellent results with Performance Massage and hope that you will find it equally rewarding.

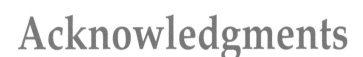

# Acknowledgments

*I*t gives me great pleasure to publicly acknowledge all of the people who helped make this book possible. I am grateful to April Parker, Patricia Meltzer, and Carol Smalley for their assistance in clarifying, typing, and organizing the text. A special thanks goes to Nancy Dail and Linda Jaros Osga for their support and assistance in this project.

I am also indebted to the entire staff at Human Kinetics. Special thanks go to Rainer Martens for his ongoing support of this book and to Holly Gilly for her skill and patience as my developmental editor.

I am appreciative of the students and faculty at the Chicago School of Massage Therapy for their ongoing feedback, input, and insight. I am indeed fortunate to be part of such an innovative and supportive professional training center.

To the members and officers of the American Massage Therapy Association, I extend a special thank-you. Their support and contributions to the advancement of the profession have set the stage for dramatic public acceptance of this craft.

I am especially indebted to Leon Chaitow, Therese Forsthoefel, and David Lauterstein for their expertise, compassion, and positive impact on my professional development. Their influence certainly transcends technical expertise. I appreciate their embodiment of the values and vision of the natural healing arts.

And finally I give my heartfelt thanks to my wife, Kathie, for her loyalty, support, and belief in this project. As always, her support has been invaluable.

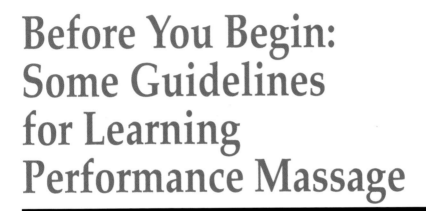

# Before You Begin: Some Guidelines for Learning Performance Massage

*P*erformance Massage is a relative newcomer to fitness, dance, and athletic training programs. Previous books on the subject, especially those written for the performers themselves and not for athletic trainers, are few. Before you add Performance Massage to your activity program (or help others add it to theirs), we need to cover a few bases.

This introduction first clears up some of the common misconceptions you may have about massage therapy and then explains specifically how to use this book to learn Performance Massage and implement it in your fitness or training program.

## Some Common Massage Misconceptions

The art and science of massage therapy is often misunderstood by health care professionals and the public alike. Although sport and fitness communities are far more knowledgeable now than in recent years, some misconceptions about the practice of therapeutic massage still prevail. Let's set the record straight on some of these!

### I'm Not Strong Enough to Practice Massage

If you think you aren't strong enough to practice massage, you're probably wrong. Some of the best massage practitioners weigh no more than 110 pounds and possess only average strength. The key to their (and your) effectiveness is employing the appropriate leverage, body mechanics, and hand positioning. Once you learn the essential components of body mechanics outlined in Chapter 4, you will be able to practice Performance Massage efficiently and without fatigue.

### Massage Must Be Boring— Having to Give the Same Routine Over and Over

The misconception that practicing massage is boring is probably based on the assumption that massage therapists use the same formula and format for all recipients. Nothing could be farther from the truth. Contemporary professional therapists are challenged to be creative, intuitive, and willing to change their treatment strategies on an ongoing basis. No two people are the same. A thin, 110-pound recreational runner requires different applications of massage than a 300-pound lineman in professional football. By developing your sensitivity and intuitive skills, you will be able to personalize your Performance Massage session to the needs of the person you're working with.

### My Hands Will Get Too Tired From Doing Massage

One of the most common fallacies about massage is believing your hands will get tired. At our school in Chicago and in workshops I teach, a major theme is the correct use of hand and arm biomechanics.

Many of us remember massaging a parent or family member when we were young. Our massage "technique" was to squeeze or knead until our hands hurt. We probably also had cramping in the forearms and general fatigue in the arms and shoulders. The key to avoiding hand and arm strain is to vary the application of techniques and implement proper biomechanics. In Performance Massage, the hands are seldom, if ever, overused, because hand positioning is continually changing.

## Reading and Practicing the Techniques in This Book Will Enable Me to Become a Professional Massage Therapist

Massage therapy today is an emerging profession with accredited schools, a national certification program, and an evolving scope of practice. In many states the profession is regulated by licensure. Our intent in teaching Performance Massage is to bring massage to the exercising public to enhance fitness and sport participation. Charging fees for a session is not advised unless you have completed the appropriate "initiation rites" into the profession. This would include graduation from an accredited school with a thorough understanding of anatomy, physiology, kinesiology, pathology, theory and practice of massage, and several different technique applications. Appendix A lists some resources that will be helpful to you if you decide to continue your education and pursue a professional career in this field. In the meantime, continue to practice and master Performance Massage; a profound, highly-developed sense of touch, coupled with fundamental hands-on skills, is one of the most useful and interesting talents you can acquire for performing massage.

## Popping the Neck and Cracking the Back Are Acceptable in the Practice of Massage

Wrong! If you apply thrusting manipulations to the bones, you are no longer practicing massage therapy. Manipulative forms of health care, such as chiropractic and osteopathy, sometimes employ these techniques, but they are well beyond the intent or scope of this book. I personally believe that if you take care to normalize the muscles and connective tissues of the body, adjustment techniques will seldom be necessary. In fact, many practitioners of manipulative medicine are now employing soft-tissue approaches as part of a holistic program of structural alignment and body maintenance. Let safety and service be your overriding intent as you practice Performance Massage.

## Massage Is a Medical Specialty and Should Be Practiced Only By Physical Therapists and Physicians

Massage therapy today is practiced with peak performance athletes, in hospital delivery rooms, as part of athletic rehabilitation, at chronic pain centers, and at most health clubs and spas. It is not uncommon to find psychologists, physical therapists, nurses, priests, sociologists, ministers, and exercise physiologists pursuing professional training in massage to supplement their practices or possibly as a second career. Massage therapy is probably best practiced by massage therapists, who have specific training in the field. Most health care providers receive very little, if any, formal massage training.

Certainly some forms of massage are therapeutic, such as working on scar tissue and postoperative techniques. However, in this book we emphasize prevention, wellness, and health enhancement. These techniques can be learned by most everyone and understood and practiced as educational, developmental, or family practice skills.

When I began practicing massage 20 years ago, the common stereotype was that masseurs were broken-down prize-fighters wearing sleeveless T-shirts who hacked, beat, and pummeled on the clients' backs. Masseuses were usually considered insensitive practitioners whose techniques caused their clients to wince and beg for mercy. I would like to think that our culture has become more educated in the ensuing years, but the notion that massage therapy can be sensitive and gentle is still a new idea for many people.

As these lingering misconceptions continue to fade, they will be supplanted by themes of personal wellness and relaxation, overall body care, and a dictum of the ancient Greeks: "Know thyself!"

Most athletes and physically active people suffer from mechanical stress, pain, and overuse syndromes. I have designed a total-body approach to massage to ensure optimal wellness and high-level performance. Having practiced massage in health clubs, spas, at the finish lines of major marathons, in hospitals, and at pain treatment centers, I know that by receiving skilled massage therapy, people can generally feel better, have more energy, heal faster, have improved blood circulation, and possess a more profound acceptance of their bodies.

By developing an expertise in Performance Massage, you too can make a difference.

## How to Use This Book

Because you're reading this book, I assume that you're interested in using Performance Massage to enhance your fitness, dance, or athletic training program and ultimately your performance. As you get into the heart of the book, however, you'll notice that you are taught to *give* Performance Massage. The logical question is, How will knowing how to *do* Performance Massage improve my fitness or my artistic or athletic performance?

The answer is that the best way to get the most out of this book is to use it with a training partner and perform the Performance Massage techniques on each other. You will each gain the benefits that massage brings, and, not incidentally, you will also gain the satisfaction of knowing that you're helping others.

*Performance Massage* is divided into six chapters. The first introduces you to Performance Massage, explaining what it is and what makes it unique. Chapter 2 tells you how Performance Massage can help you in your fitness or athletic training program. The third chapter describes when it's appropriate to use Performance Massage and when it's not. It also includes guidelines for Warm-Up, Cool-Down, and Maintenance Massage. Chapter 4 teaches you the basic skills you need for giving and getting a Performance Massage, and chapter 5 teaches you the specific techniques you'll use in Performance Massage. In the last chapter you'll find an entire head-to-toe Performance Massage sequence you can use to practice the techniques you've learned.

You'll find two appendixes at the end of the book. The first provides names and addresses of resources you can contact, if you're interested in purchasing some massage equipment or learning more about massage. The second illustrates the bones and major muscles of the body. Refer to this appendix as you're learning the techniques, to help you enhance their therapeutic impact.

I believe Performance Massage is a significant addition to any physical fitness or athletic training program. It is my sincere hope that, after you've learned the techniques, performed them, and received the benefits of having them applied to you, you'll share that belief.

## Chapter 1

# Introducing Performance Massage

*P*erformance Massage is different from mainstream massage, which usually consists of a generalized relaxation sequence applied with a lubricant and long, slow, connecting strokes called "effleurage." Performance Massage also differs from the specialized forms of medical massage, which are injury-specific and use deep (and sometimes painful), anatomically precise techniques.

## What Performance Massage Is

Performance Massage is the application of creative and intuitive touching skills to enhance expressive movement and athletic performance. Performance Massage includes some of the technical variations of classical massage but directs them toward a human body that is engaged in regular physical activity, dance, or on-going athletic endeavors. In this way it is a skill system whose mission is to support, encourage, and complement integrative and expressive movement.

## Ten Features That Make Performance Massage Unique

Performance Massage is characterized by the following unique features:

- The fundamental techniques can be learned by anyone.
- Clothing stays on, making massage more accessible to the athlete.
- No skin lubricant is needed.
- It is designed for athletes and other physically active people.
- It can be employed before or after activity and as part of a regular maintenance program.
- It is of shorter duration than most massage—performed in 30 minutes or less.
- It encourages intuition and creativity in its application.
- It features therapeutic stretching as a complement to massage techniques.
- It encourages an integrative, whole-body experience.
- Performance Massage is user-friendly—it feels great!

Let's take a look at each of these characteristics.

### The Fundamentals Can Be Learned By Anyone

The actual skills employed in massage are not difficult, and they can be learned quickly by anyone who is willing to practice regularly. Touch is instinctive to all of us. However, it is also a skill that requires practice, good judgment, and creativity. *Performance Massage* supports the development of a profound and positive sense of touch.

### Clothing Stays On

Most forms of massage are received in the nude while one is draped with sheets and towels. This is appropriate for Swedish massage and relaxation approaches, but Performance Massage is different. The clothing need not be removed, because the techniques involve direct pressure to the layering of muscle tissue beneath the skin. There is no need for superficial gliding over the surface of the skin. Also, the vast array of muscle-stretching techniques involved make it impractical for the recipient to be nude and covered with sheets and towels.

The fact that clothes stay on during Performance Massage makes massage more accessible. You can provide sessions in training rooms, on-site at some sporting events, in some locker rooms, backstage at a concert hall, or in an area that you and a training partner set aside. Performance Massage can be performed through a bathing suit, running shorts, leotards, or even a sweatsuit.

The fact that clothes stay on may also reassure those who are touch-sensitive or concerned about modesty. The recipient can more fully relax while you are performing the massage. As you can well imagine, it is often not practical to remove clothing before or after an athletic event, performance, or workout. When I provide Cool-Down Massage with athletes at events such as marathons or triathlons, I like to consider whatever clothing they are wearing just another layer of skin to be worked through in addressing the deeper muscles.

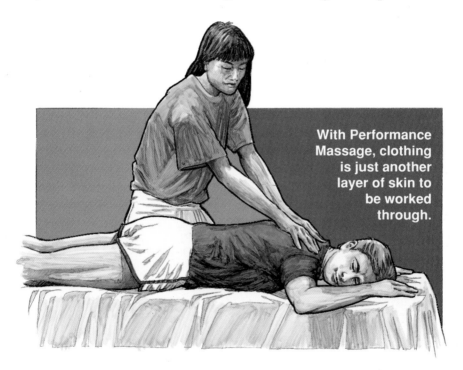

With Performance Massage, clothing is just another layer of skin to be worked through.

## No Skin Lubricant is Needed

It is not necessary to apply oil or any other skin lubricant in the recipient-centered approach of Performance Massage. This is because the effleurage stroke is not employed. Instead we stimulate circulation and warm the tissue through the various compression techniques outlined in chapter 5.

Avoiding the use of oil makes the session more practical, for the recipient won't need to use astringents or shower afterward to remove a greasy or oily residue. Also, Performance Massage, by virtue of clothing being on, uses a series of grasps and techniques not dependent on effleurage or strokes requiring a lubricant.

## Designed for Athletes and Active People

Performance Massage lengthens and decongests the muscles, tendons, and other connective tissues of the body by employing a creative combination of high-impact massage techniques along with muscle stretching. This approach encourages greater flexibility, enhanced motion, and overall body mobility, which are essential for peak performance.

## Can Be Used Before or After Activity and As Maintenance

When the musculature is kept in an optimal physiological state, many common injuries and the all-too-familiar aches and pains of exertion can be minimized. A Warm-Up Massage can be developed for use before physical exertion. A Cool-Down Massage is also an effective therapeutic measure after exercise. Performed on an ongoing basis, Maintenance Massage can set the stage for activity at full capacity.

## Shorter Than Most Massage Sessions

Because our approach is devoid of superficial or accessory massage strokes, it can easily be performed in 30 minutes or less. This suits the temperament of active people, most of whom would find 60- or 90-minute sessions to be too long. By performing a 30-minute, up-tempo, and rhythmic massage, you can reach your objectives of muscle unwinding and circulatory stimulation without compromising quality.

## Encourages Intuition and Creativity in Its Application

Very often traditional massage is learned and practiced as a generic sequence. Although this may be appropriate for some recipients, many others will find it to be a lethargic, mechanical hands-on experience. Performance Massage is different. You will be learning specific techniques, but you will also be encouraged to use your hands as sensors, feeling the tissues for areas of tension. By doing this, you can personalize your session and focus on specific problem areas for each individual.

Intuition is a capacity that we all possess. By using your hands intuitively, you will notice that your techniques blend with one another. Professional therapists often note that massage becomes an art form when these subtleties are blended into a comprehensive and creative session. Also, the specific techniques become much less intimidating when you feel confident that you already have a well-developed sense of touch.

## Features Therapeutic Stretching

By incorporating muscle-stretching movements with your hands-on techniques, you can focus your attention on creating a uniquely therapeutic session. Specifically, you can lengthen the muscles that feel taut, thereby enhancing flexibility and range of motion. This can complement a warm-up, and it feels especially good after the strain and stress of physical exertion.

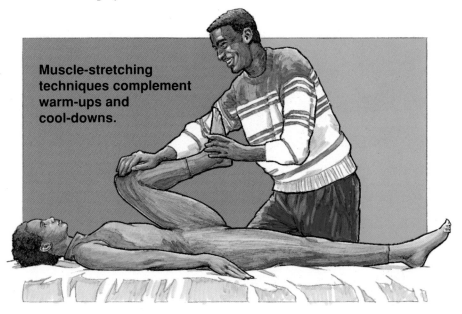

Muscle-stretching techniques complement warm-ups and cool-downs.

## Encourages an Integrative, Whole-Body Experience

Much mainstream massage is performed technique by technique, sequence by sequence. This can give the recipient a feeling of being fragmented. Performance Massage, particularly through its use of compression, allows you to work on two areas of the musculature at the same time. By applying leverage and pressure simultaneously, you can begin to unwind or unknot the musculature and create a sense of wholeness or totality. Soft tissues soften, lengthen, and assume more pliability from massage. Because movement is a total process, this is an important concept and one that will not be lost on the recipient.

## It's User-Friendly

Painful muscular aches, injuries, and soreness can produce a negative psychological disposition. It is important to experience the body in a positive and self-accepting fashion. Performance Massage is the key in making this vital connection. It feels good, both during and after, so prepare to become very popular as you practice and master the essentials of Performance Massage.

# Chapter 2

# Performance Massage: Just Right for Active People

*T*hose who are highly motivated to be active, whether professional quarterbacks, performing artists, or "weekend warriors" entering a 10-mile run, often subject their bodies to extraordinary stresses, strains, and demands. Competitive athletes, weekend warriors, dancers, and even participants in rigorous fitness programs are usually committed to maximum effort, faster times, and peak performance. Along with the tremendous increase in physical fitness and sport participation in recent years, there has been a corresponding increase in the number of strain and overuse injuries.

## Special Needs of Active People

If you are to make a genuine contribution to the athletic, fitness, or training programs of the people you intend to massage, it would seem useful to understand common reasons why those involved

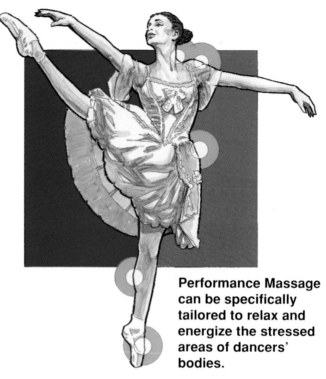

**Performance Massage can be specifically tailored to relax and energize the stressed areas of dancers' bodies.**

in such programs are injured and spend much downtime recovering from injuries. The following are the major causes of activity-related injuries.

## Lack of Circulation

Active people use their muscles more than those who are inactive, which means their muscles need more blood and nutrients to nourish them than do the muscles of sedentary people. Increased physical activity strengthens the body's circulatory mechanisms but can also be a source of dysfunction. Excessive repetitive motion can cause a tightening of muscles and soft tissues, blocking the normal circulatory flow of blood to that area. Additionally, metabolic wastes and toxins can become embedded in tissue, resulting in a state of toxicity that impedes peak performance.

## Tight Muscles

Muscles often become excessively tight, and this can affect flexibility, relaxation, and muscle balance. Tight muscles result from overuse, excessive stress, and the accumulative wear and tear on tissue that is unable to withstand continual overload. Some of the common pains due to tightening include pain in the jaw muscles, which often tense in a clenching of the teeth during maximum exertion; pain in the temples, resulting from exhaustion, overtraining, or poor breathing mechanics; pain in the back of the neck, resulting from a forward head tilt, poor posture, or prevailing anxiety; pain in upper back muscles, resulting from muscular tension, postural slouching, or rounded shoulders; low back pain from unequal leg length, pelvic rotation, or generalized stress or anxiety; or buttock pain, which can also occur in leg-length discrepancy, a rotated pelvis, or overuse of one leg (such as running on uneven surfaces). Hands often manifest tension through clenching and squeezing—typical of the person with a high competitive drive or one who is overly zealous and high-strung. The muscle attachments and soft tissues around the knee can be overstressed from sudden stopping, bracing, or twisting or from movements occurring while off-balance. The tendons and ligaments of the ankle are commonly stressed through uneven weight distribution, sudden twisting of the foot, or repetitive movements on uneven surfaces. Abdominal discomfort can stem from nervous tension, shallow breathing, or chronic nervousness. Even the soles of the feet can reflect tension, from clenching or curling of the toes, inappropriate footwear, or overly flexible flat feet.

All of these conditions can distort or disturb physical integrity, and cause postural compensation that can result in chronic pain.

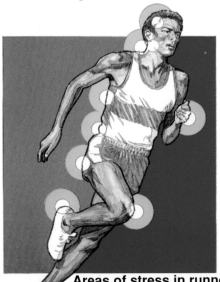

**Areas of stress in runners that result in chronic pain can be helped by Performance Massage.**

## Injuries

Active people sometimes get injured. Perhaps the most common cause of physical breakdown is the "too much, too soon" syndrome, where physical makeup is simply insufficient for the intensity of the chosen activity. For instance, a runner who increases his or her training schedule from 10 to 22 miles during the period of a week will likely incur a series of overuse syndromes, such as burnout, fatigue, unresolved aches and pains, and slight tearing of connective tissues. Other factors that contribute to activity-related injuries include muscle imbalance, inadequate warm-up, poor flexibility, mineral deficiency, structural abnormality, lack of endurance, and reoccurrence of previous injuries.

## Muscle Soreness

Active people's muscles get sore, and this inhibits activity and performance. There are many theories regarding muscle soreness, but one of the most commonly accepted is that of microscopic tearing in connective tissues as a result of repeated demands on a particular part of the body. These repetitive stresses and contractions can lead to tearing, cellular inflammation, and pain as the muscles shorten, splint, and bind together in a protective reaction. Obviously, if someone continues to "work through" the soreness under an ill-advised application of the "no pain, no gain" motto, she or he simply sets the physiological stage for further injury and breakdown.

## Scarring and Adhesions in Soft Tissues

Adhesions and scar tissues sometimes form on soft tissues and affect muscle integrity and range of motion. As these unresolved, seemingly minor aches and pains continue to be stressed by exertion, more significant injuries occur, leading to chronic pain and a degeneration in the body's soft tissues. *Adhesions* are unhealed tissues that often mat, adhere, or stick together. They may also become glued onto ligaments, other tissues, or bones. If adhesions are not properly treated, they can become chronic and form an immobile scar that permanently reduces range of motion.

Unresolved scar tissues embedded in key postural muscles produces a myofascial drag on the body (a restriction of muscles and fascia), wastes enormous energy, and often results in mediocre performance. Even more important, the stage is now set for frequent recurrence of injury.

## Mind/Body Connection

Optimal physical output is often described by active people as a "coming together" of all body parts, where motion itself becomes relaxed, integrated, and even effortless. The person with a keen self-awareness will be able to identify, even pinpoint, the location of pain, inflammation, or restriction preventing total body involvement in the kinetic symphony of performance. This kinesthetic sense of feeling, listening to, and trusting the body not only provides a psychological boost—it also helps to prevent injuries and overuse.

"Know thyself," said the ancient Greeks. A developed self-awareness will enhance the inherent poise and poetry of high-level physical functioning.

Self-awareness often overlaps with self-esteem and self-confidence. The person who feels better on a gut level will often perform better. Performance Massage will not replace systematic activity or sport conditioning; it does, however, complement it. The person "in touch" will be able to better withstand the extraordinary physical demands on the body. This "competitive edge" often separates excellent from good performance and high-level output from the performance slump.

# How Performance Massage Meets the Needs of Active People

Performance Massage is tailor-made to serve the needs of athletes and other fitness enthusiasts. It provides benefits that are particularly suited to the stresses and strains of athletic or movement training and performance or a regular fitness program.

- It improves the circulation of blood and lymph, helping to maintain the muscles and soft tissues in an optimum state of nutrition.
- It reduces muscle tightness and restriction, creating improved tone, flexibility, and relaxation as well as promoting overall muscle balance.
- It enables the recipient to recover more rapidly from injury and reduces the likelihood of further injury.
- It reduces muscle soreness, enabling more consistent, higher-level training and performance.
- Cross-fiber massage effectively reduces adhesions and some degrees of scar tissue formation in the soft tissues. This allows for restoration of muscle integrity and full range of motion.

- It reduces pain and promotes overall relaxation.
- It helps to enhance body awareness—assisting in fully expressive movement.
- It provides a psychological boost and generates self-confidence.

*Chapter 3*

# When to Use Performance Massage

By now I hope I've convinced you of how beneficial Performance Massage can be—and made you eager to incorporate it into your training routine or fitness program or to help others incorporate it into theirs. I'll spend the next few pages discussing how to schedule massage sessions, when Performance Massage should *not* be used, and how to effectively incorporate it into a training and competition schedule.

## Scheduling Massage Sessions

Anyone who is committed to her or his sport, fitness program, or art form will find Performance Massage indispensable to the attainment of fitness and performance goals. Ideally, Performance Massage should be experienced daily, before or after workouts. If this is not possible, try to utilize this unique approach at least twice a week for

20 minutes to assure cumulative and ongoing results. For physical and psychological benefits, once a week is the absolute minimum to receive massage. As active people continue to use Performance Massage, the stretching movements become easier, flexibility is enhanced, and the muscles become more pliable and receptive to touch.

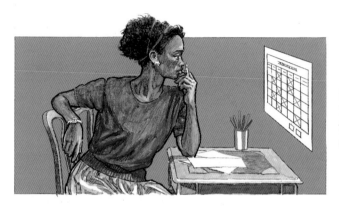

**Use Performance Massage at least twice a week for optimal results.**

Plan massage sessions carefully to ensure that a regular fitness habit is being implemented. For each massage session, allow ample time to apply the techniques systematically and thoroughly. Remember, a massage session needs to be a time of relaxation, unwinding, nonverbal communication, and physical and psychological reduction of stress. This certainly cannot be achieved if you have one eye on the hamstrings and the other one on your watch!

## Precautions for Performance Massage

Touch, in and of itself, is healing. It has a positive effect on the skin, the circulation, and many vital organs and systems of the body. Because massage is a healing art, knowing what to do and what not to do is as important as knowing what you are capable of doing. Good judgment is as important as any of the skills you master from reading this book.

If you are uncertain about anything regarding a recipient's physical condition, do not administer massage. Play it safe. If you have any questions, seek the advice of a qualified medical practitioner before commencing your session. Remember, the objective of Performance Massage is injury prevention and enhanced movement, so be certain that you are not attempting to diagnose or treat a specific medical condition.

At times you may need to modify your session because of certain medical conditions. There is one general rule for Performance Massage: when in doubt, don't. This approach will assure that physiological limitations are being respected.

The Greek physician Hippocrates perhaps summed it up best, several millenia ago, when he said, "Above all, do no harm." When the following conditions are present, do not use Performance Massage.

■ *Do not massage when tissues are inflamed.* Inflammation is part of the body's defense and healing process that takes place when tissue has been damaged or injured. It is the body's attempt to isolate damaged tissue and protect it from further injuries. These are the five signs of inflammation:

—Redness from increased blood flow to the body part
—Heat, also resulting from increased blood flow to a localized area
—Swelling, due to increased cellular activity and blood engorgement
—Pain, due to the release of the chemical histamine and the increased pressure of cellular fluids on local nerves
—Loss of movement, resulting from excitation of the nervous system, contraction of the musculature, and increased fluid accumulation

■ *Do not massage when severe pain is present in joints, bones, or muscles.* These symptoms may indicate sprains, fractures, or other conditions well beyond the scope of your massage session.

■ *Never put pressure on swollen or painful joints.* Conditions such as bursitis and arthritis can be exacerbated by inappropriate massage. Keep communication lines open with the recipient so that you are not inadvertently aggravating an arthritic or chronic joint condition.

■ *Be cautious with people in the advanced stages of diabetes.* Advanced stages of diabetes often involve severe disturbances in circulation, which are characterized by edema and swelling of the joints. Deep pressure can cause tissue damage, so individuals should check with a physician prior to receiving a massage.

■ *Do not massage cancerous areas, tumors, or cysts.* If you are in doubt about a particular lesion, play it safe and stay away from the area. Recipients should consult with a physician regarding any abnormal growth or tumor.

■ *Massage should not be applied if the recipient has a contagious illness or an elevated temperature.* Flu, colds, and certain other viruses leave the person weak. Massage can often cause nausea at these times.

■ *Do not massage directly on open wounds or burns.*

■ *Do not massage directly on any rashes or skin infections.* A localized rash, however, in most cases will not prohibit you from working on other parts of the body.

■ *Do not apply direct pressure over varicose veins.*

■ *Do not massage areas where blood clots or phlebitis* (inflamed blood vessels) *have occurred.* A medical profile can assist in the exercise of good judgment.

■ *Use caution on people with some cardiac conditions, such as a recent heart attack or excessively high, untreated blood pressure.* The heart may not tolerate the increased stimulation from deep massage. However, athletes and physically active people who control their blood pressure with medication may be massaged. Limiting the duration of a session to 15 minutes and utilizing light pressure are good precautions.

■ *Do not massage a person who is feeling physically ill.* Anyone with symptoms such as nausea, shivering, or excess cramping due to hyper- or hypothermia should be referred to medical personnel. Such symptoms are common at the finish line of major marathons

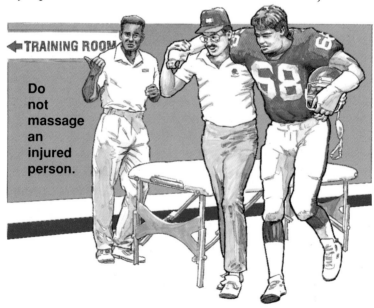

and triathlons, and the athlete should be referred to a primary care health provider.

Our objectives are to relieve the tension, movement restrictions, and soreness often caused by the abuse, overuse, and misuse of the body during physical exertion. By keeping your objectives for Performance Massage simple and safe, you will rarely encounter any serious problems. Knowing when to refer to a physician is characteristic of a caring and competent practitioner.

Above all, remember that massage is adjunctive to medical care. Be sure you are not taking on the role of a doctor. Diagnosis of any medical condition is beyond your expertise and existing legal parameters. Be realistic about your massage intentions and objectives. Be clear that your session is not designed to treat a specific disease or to fix a complicated structural misalignment. Know the benefits as well as the limitations of your session. Always keep in mind that massage is a healing art. Practicing good judgment is as essential as any of the skills you master in this book.

If, though, people are healthy, there's no reason they can't benefit from Performance Massage before a workout or competition, after a workout or competition, or as a maintenance activity. I explain in the massage technique descriptions in chapter 5 which of the techniques are best suited for use in Warm-Up and Cool-Down massage sessions.

## Warm-Up Massage

Massage before exercise, performance, or competition is given as an adjunct to, but not a substitute for, the physical warm-up. Massaging before exercise or an athletic or artistic event has physiological and psychological benefits.

### Goals of Warm-Up Massage

Warm-Up Performance Massage creates a state of readiness within the muscles and tissues by stimulating circulation and generating a fresh, abundant supply of oxygenated blood to an area. This is known as hyperemia.

Massage also helps the muscles to work longer and become more efficient by reducing tension and increasing the flexibility of tight muscle groups. It can enhance the general state of well-being, thereby assisting in relaxation, focused concentration, centering, and visualization techniques.

## Warm-Up Massage Guidelines

Massage before an event or exercise should be light, of short duration, nonspecific, and warming. Emphasis should be placed on the muscles to be used for the particular activity. The pace is up-tempo and rhythmic, to simultaneously relax and energize. Be certain that your session does not include any painful or high-impact techniques. Deep cross-fiber friction would not be recommended just prior to exercising. Also take care that you do not overwork the muscle or relax the recipient to the point where he or she becomes sleepy or unfocused.

For these reasons it is best to apply a 15- to 20-minute Warm-Up Massage prior to exercise or an event. Ideally this should be done 30 to 45 minutes before the event, as an adjunct to the actual warm-up. However, this will often depend on the event itself, weather conditions, practical considerations, and whether you own a portable table.

Be sure you take into account the recipient's familiarity with massage. A person's responses may depend on his or her past experiences with massage and their overall familiarity with your sense of touch. In his book *Winning Triathlon*, Scott Tinley, one of the world's greatest triathletes, describes the overall value of massage as well as the caution that should be taken by those less familiar with massage therapy.

"By no means get your first massage the day before an important competition. I learned that lesson the hard way before the Iron Man in 1982. A big Hawaiian woman gave me her $25 special, and I woke up the next morning feeling as if I had been run over by a truck."

Also remember that athletes and artists are often ritualistic, eccentric, and highly idiosyncratic just before an event or performance; their last-minute behavior may simply not accommodate being massaged. Acknowledge this boundary.

In time, bodies will come to "accept a massage," and the recipient will learn to relax individual muscle groups during a massage. As your massage sessions progress over time, your fingers will glide over muscle fibers that they were struggling through only a month before.

## The Psychological Edge

There is fine-tuning involved in getting psyched for competition or performance whether it's a workout at the gym, dancing in your first recital, or a Sunday-afternoon game of touch football. If the individual is to perform to the best of her or his ability, it is essential that physical capacity and mental focusing become synchronized. Performance Massage assists in experiencing a synchronized body-mind experience prior to exertion. It

- provides quality downtime in which to mentally focus on the impending event;
- provides relaxation and anxiety reduction, allowing enhanced performance to occur naturally;
- provides a pre-event ritual consistent with many performers' idiosyncrasies;
- flushes and oxygenates the muscles, creating the physiological environment for optimal performance;
- initiates a powerful effect, enhancing the competitive edge; and
- provides an opportunity to practice meditation or visualization techniques conducive to excellence.

A highly anxious, hypertense person obviously needs to be calmed down or relaxed during the Warm-Up Massage session. This allows the recipient to become more focused and avoid diffusing psychic energy through random nervousness. Your techniques need to be slow and rhythmic, creating a near-hypnotic effect on the high-strung person. You can also focus on breathing techniques and gentle stretching to facilitate the recipient's experience of weightless and free movement. The tenor and resonance of your voice is also important for guiding the recipient to the optimal performance state.

The opposite applies to the lethargic or poorly motivated person. Your techniques need to be more up-tempo and energizing, with emphasis on muscle flushing and energy movements. This quickened approach can be complemented by inspirational or motivational dialogue if it seems appropriate. Also, extra hand pressure can create a sense of exhilaration vital to the intricate process of getting psyched.

Whatever the person's disposition, be conscious of your role in producing the physical and psychological centeredness that often separates maximum effort from a mediocre performance.

## Warm-Up Massage Summary

To summarize, the goals of Performance Massage before exercise or performance are to

- relax tight muscle groups;
- increase flexibility and range of motion;
- decrease anxiety and nervous tension;
- increase circulation, allowing muscles to work longer and more efficiently;
- enhance psychological preparedness concurrent with focusing or visualization techniques; and
- create a unified, whole-body experience.

Remember these guidelines as you prepare for a Warm-Up Performance Massage.

- No deep pressure or highly specific work such as cross-fiber friction.
- Keep the session to 20 minutes or less.
- Keep a rhythmic and up-beat pace.
- Work lightly.

Be conservative in applying massage before exercise, so that you don't overdo it, and be sure to avoid working on areas of the body that are recovering from injury. This applies to massage not only right before an event or exercise but even a day or two prior to an event requiring maximum performance. By practicing this conservative approach and utilizing the Warm-Up Massage as an adjunct and not as a "last-minute secret weapon," you can take a more intelligent approach to working with the athlete, performer, or fitness enthusiast on a long-term basis.

## Cool-Down Massage

Performance Massage is beneficial after athletic competition, artistic performance, or a  challenging workout. It promotes a general state of relaxation, helps reduce lingering muscle tension, and can help eliminate subsequent muscular soreness. It will also help the muscles recover more quickly from fatigue. The length of recovery time from exertion can also be significantly reduced with a good postevent session.

### Goals of Cool-Down Massage

The goal of your Cool-Down Performance Massage after exertion is similar to that of your session prior to exertion—you mainly want to assist circulation and stretch tightened muscles. The physiological condition of the recipient, however, is now quite different.

After exercise the muscles are in a state of congestion and fatigue, particularly following maximum exertion. The tissues and muscles are filled with metabolic wastes, and circulatory assistance is needed for the elimination of these wastes. Therefore the circulatory techniques of compression, flushing, and energy movements will be particularly effective in restoring balance and equilibrium.

## Cool-Down Massage Guidelines

When applying massage after exertion, be attentive to the tone and sensitivity of the recipient's muscles, which may differ greatly from their previous session. Be sure that your pressure does not cause any pain, and be aware that some muscles may be unduly sensitive to your touch. So gauge your pressure accordingly, and massage gradually, with the intent of loosening and decongesting the musculature.

Keep in mind that the sooner you are able to perform the Cool-Down Massage session, the more effective your techniques will be. Ideally massage should be done shortly after exertion as part of the cool-down process. This will help the recipient physically and psychologically unwind from the stresses and strains of maximum exertion.

Although massaging through running shorts, leotards, or even sweat pants should present no problem, do help the recipient remove his or her shoes, especially after a lengthy workout, as this can be painful for an inflexible person.

As a safety precaution, ask the following questions to assure that your session can be performed without unnecessary risk:

- How are you feeling?
- Would you like something to drink?
- What physical areas need particular attention?
- Are you feeling hot, warm, cold? Is everything OK?
- Keep me posted on any technique that feels good or let me know if it's too much pressure.

Try to have water available for the recipient immediately after exercising. This will prevent dehydration, which can be extremely harmful. If for any reason you feel the recipient may have been injured or exceeded training and workout limitations, it is advisable to refer to a primary health care provider such as an athletic trainer, a dance coach, or a sports medicine specialist.

Know the symptoms of hyperthermia (excessive body temperature). They include

- excessive sweating,
- shivering or chilling,
- dry skin,
- nausea,
- a throbbing pressure in the head,
- an unsteady gait,
- lack of focus,
- extreme fatigue, and
- excessive cramping.

If you observe any of these symptoms, have the recipient lie down, give fluids, and seek medical help. Do not apply massage, because this could add to unsteadiness, nausea, or fatigue.

During cold weather, have the recipient take a warm shower and thoroughly loosen and relax the body before you administer massage. Provided it is dry, sweat clothing should be kept on to prevent chilling or unnecessary stiffening of the muscles.

Keep your Cool-Down Massage to 20 minutes or less. Keep your session balanced, but if there is an area of tension or stiffness, you may wish to devote extra attention to these problem areas. You can do this by applying compression variations and gentle muscle stretching.

## Cool-Down Massage as a Reward

In performing sports massage at races and athletic events across the country, I frequently hear athletes exclaim that the only reason they enter a particular race or athletic event is because they know the American Massage Therapy Association Sports Massage Team will be at the finish line. Massage is also its own reward. Athletes, performers, and physically fit people are often highly motivated, sometimes excessively so, in their pursuit of achievement. Although achievement may be its own reward, it nevertheless is good psychology to reinforce and encourage the attainment of secondary or sequential goals along the way. Applying massage in conjunction with the achievement of performance success only reinforces the positive and health-enhancing nature of your session.

For instance, when a dancer performs a routine perfectly after days of rehearsal, or when an aerobic dance-class participant's resting heart rate drops after a month of working out, a significant

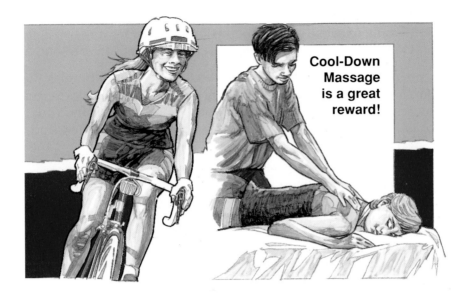

Cool-Down Massage is a great reward!

performance level is achieved. This would be an ideal time to schedule the massage session. Sometimes the additional stress on the body and mind, as well as the repetitive impact of increased training, will make a person especially receptive to and appreciative of massage benefits.

Keep in mind that massage may be an important motivating factor for obtaining a new level of fitness or performance. Both physically and psychologically, the massage experience should be harmonious with maximum performance.

## Cool-Down Massage Summary

To summarize, the goals of Performance Massage after exercise are to

- assist in the cool-down process,
- provide general relief from exhaustion,
- relax tight muscle groups,
- stimulate circulation, and
- reduce potential soreness.

Remember these guidelines as you prepare for a Cool-Down Performance Massage:

- Be temperature-conscious in regard to overheating and chilling.
- Have water available.

- ■ Be gentle! Realize that the recipient may be physically or emotionally exhausted, and keep your pressure light.
- ■ Do not massage if symptoms of hyperthermia are present.

A benefit of massage after exercise is that it promotes relaxation from the strains and overuse that often occur with physical exertion. The recipient will feel better physically and psychologically. You can also help reduce those nagging aches and pains that often lead to major injuries.

## Maintenance Massage

A person does not need to experience the painful stresses and strains of overuse in order to enjoy the benefits of Performance Massage. Maintenance Massage is regularly scheduled, weekly or twice-weekly sessions designed to maintain peak operating condition. It is not unlike regular tuneups for your car. By applying Performance Massage within the framework of overall body maintenance, you can help prevent overuse injuries, enhance endurance by keeping the muscles performing longer, and ultimately prolong the recipient's career.

Massage before and after exercise is abbreviated and adjunctive to the warm-up and cool-down processes. The major impact of Maintenance Massage is obtained by the regular, ongoing, cumulative changes in the tissues. This is why regular, ongoing, twice-weekly sessions will produce a regenerative effect, prevent injuries, and keep the body in optimal condition.

Maintenance Massage must be performed at least once a week to ensure therapeutic results. Ideally this can be scheduled at a regular time each week to encourage massage as being an essential component of a training regime. I have found good results utilizing massage on the rest day. This way you can avoid the concerns of pre- and postexercise massage and instead concentrate on performing a comprehensive 30-minute session.

# Chapter 4

# Preparing for Performance Massage

*P*erformance Massage is easily added to a dance or athletic training program or workout schedule. Little equipment is needed, and the basic techniques are easy to learn and deliver. Some preparation is required, however, for maximum benefit. This chapter describes how to prepare the massage environment, how to prepare yourself to give a massage, and how to prepare someone to receive a massage.

## Preparing the Massage Environment

Performance Massage can be done at almost any time or place. I have given massage sessions backstage at a dance festival, in the bleachers at Wrigley Field, at the finish line of triathlons and marathons, and even in a boxing ring between rounds. The best situation, though, is to have a comfortable place, appropriately equipped.

## Massage Area

Ideally you will want to perform your massage in an environment that is warm, relaxing, and free from noise or intrusion. I usually prefer a room that is shrouded from sunlight and without overhead lighting or harsh direct light on the face of the recipient. I find it a nice touch to have a dimmer switch to control the lighting.

Nothing can negate the beneficial effects of Performance Massage more than a chill or a draft. Cool air can cause reflexive tightening or muscle contraction. Try keeping the temperature at 72°F, or 22°C, to assure warmth.

Try to achieve a pleasant atmosphere in your massage area. Quiet background music can enhance the massage experience if the choice is acceptable to the recipient. Keep the massage area smoke-free to assure acceptable air quality. A sense of order and cleanliness should be balanced with a soft and comforting environment.

Your own appearance should contribute to the massage environment, too. I suggest you wear a short-sleeved blouse or shirt, and loose-fitting slacks let you assume the lunge position and move without restriction. Be neat and clean, and avoid strongly scented toiletries.

If you must provide Performance Massage outside of your optimal environment, such as in a dressing or training room or an area with traffic flow, consider hanging a sign asking for quiet. By anticipating any interruptions or excessive noise, you can greatly enhance receptivity to your massage.

All these tips are offered to encourage you to provide an "incubation experience" that helps the person receiving the massage unwind and experience the unifying mind/body effect of massage. By setting the stage with care, you can reassure and relax the person on the table.

## Equipment

The professional massage table is probably the most important (and expensive) tool of the trade. There are also a few other items that are nice to have around.

**Massage Table.**    Giving a massage at the side of a bed is not advisable; the mattress does not offer enough support, and you will find yourself straining your lower back. Working on the floor or on top of a mat or sleeping bag can also be difficult, as you will need to employ precise postural positioning and frequent changes of position in order to stay relaxed and comfortable. Therefore, to develop a genuine mastery of Performance Massage, purchase a table from one of the reputable companies listed in Appendix A. If you prefer, you might be able to rent a table from a local massage center or accredited massage school. Massage tables are now designed with state-of-the-art technology. They are adjustable for height and can be readily folded for transport or storage. (Incidentally, they can also be used for overnight guests, as laundry tables, or for performing stretching exercises.)

If you do not have access to a massage table, you can improvise. Most athletic locker rooms have a treatment table that can be used; or you might try a folding or kitchen table (provided it is sturdy enough) covered with 3 inches of foam rubber or, if necessary, a sleeping bag. The two main considerations when choosing a work surface are the recipient's comfort and your ability to provide massage without straining.

You might also consider building a massage table. As a general rule, the height of the table should be 3 inches below your extended arm. This will allow you to employ leverage instead of force when performing the various techniques. The dimensions of your table can vary; most professional tables are 5 feet 9 inches long and 26 inches wide.

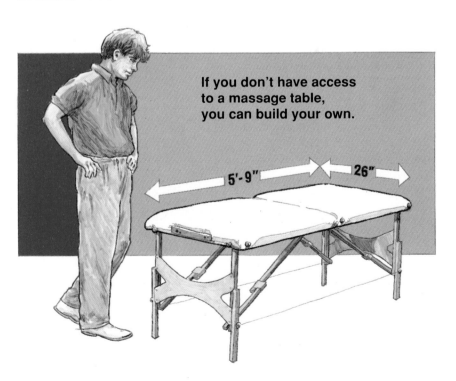

**If you don't have access to a massage table, you can build your own.**

5'-9"    26"

**Miscellaneous Equipment.**    Regardless of the surface you work on, it is a good hygienic practice to cover it with a clean sheet. Your sheet can be any color (it need not be "clinic white") and should cover the entire surface that the recipient will contact. Change sheets after each session. A supply of towels and blankets can help keep the recipient warm.

It's a nice touch to have hangers or hooks for coats, jackets, or workout apparel, and it is also helpful to have a supply of tissues, a first-aid kit, and drinking water.

Performance Massage does not require oil in its application, but you may wish to have an astringent solution such as osage rub or witch hazel to apply to the skin, especially if the recipient has just finished a workout. Astringents help close the pores and provide a tingling, refreshing feel.

A small file can hold a journal of your sessions or basic records as you chart your progress and the therapeutic results you are obtaining with the people you massage.

One final tip: You ought to wash your hands between every session, but sometimes this is not practical—such as during on-site massage at a sporting event. If you are going to be working outside or at a location where soap and water are not readily available, you might carry moist towelettes or a hand-washing antibiotic lotion that doesn't require a rinse-off.

By following these basic procedures, you can provide a safe, comfortable, hygienic session.

## Preparing Your Mind

In addition to acquiring basic massage skills, there are other specific things you can do to get yourself ready to give Performance Massage, including developing an intuitive style. More than anything else, your intent should be to have a successful session.

An integral part of providing a successful session is determining what your objectives are. I suggest that you mentally rehearse what you are trying to accomplish in your 30-minute session. Goals I establish before starting a massage session include alleviation of muscle soreness, stimulation of circulation, relaxation of taut nerve endings, unwinding of soft-tissue restrictions, and enhancement of sensory pleasure. As part of my personal preparation, I also reflect on my own potential to convey comfort, relief, and care. Think about any medical restrictions, areas of tenderness, or personal idiosyncrasies of the recipient before beginning.

Establishing these specific boundaries adds personalized clarity to your session.

The recipient's acceptance of Performance Massage may depend upon his or her age, physical condition, level of fitness, muscle soreness, and emotional poise. Taking a quick mental inventory of these factors will enable you to provide touch that is both user-friendly and highly therapeutic.

Also concentrate on the physical and emotional pleasure you will receive as you provide a session that significantly affects someone. When the person on the table emits a sigh, suddenly lets go of a tightened area, or extends a compliment regarding how good a specific stroke feels, file that compliment away in your brain, and you will find that your connection to the person and to your massage is positively enhanced. Feeling good while providing a Performance Massage, or any type of touch skill, is vital. Picture the opposite: You are standing flatfooted with locked knees, straining your back and overexerting the muscles of your arms and shoulders, with a tight jaw, clenched teeth, shallow breathing, and a prevailing sense of strain and performance anxiety. No one would enjoy such a stressful session!

Touching skills achieve a masterful state, like a peak performance experience, when there are elements of sensory knowledge, spontaneity, and that profound sense of being part of a flow that is so common to athletic peaking. Continually remind yourself that care and nurturing will sensitize your focus and hand movements.

To help yourself develop mental preparation skills, try to visualize the different massage needs of the following characters.

### ■ MENTAL EXERCISE 1 ■

Visualize a 35-year-old sedentary office worker who has spent the better part of the last 8 hours sitting in front of a video display terminal. He is tense and sluggish, has tenderness in the back of his neck and in his upper back muscles, and is probably not accustomed to being touched in a therapeutic fashion.

What would be the intent of your massage? Think through a short, 10-minute tune-up session, and let your awareness guide the subtleties of rate, rhythm, pressure, and assessment of physical tension. This form of visualization allows you to improvise to the case at hand.

### ■  MENTAL EXERCISE 2  ■

Now imagine an 84-year-old grandmother who is in frail health, gets little exercise, and often complains of headaches and nervous tension. Imagine a 5-minute session, taking into account her state of health, ability to receive pressure, and areas of stress and holding.

You probably imagined your touch being light, smooth, soft, perhaps reassuring, nurturing, and very accommodating to the physical realities of a frail and elderly person. This exercise can soften an approach that is sometimes too direct or powerful.

### ■  MENTAL EXERCISE 3  ■

Picture a 20-year-old ballet dancer who is in peak physical condition and has highly toned legs. She is used to being massaged regularly and likes deep pressure, particularly around the restrictions that develop around the hips.

Mentally shift your intent to the needs of the dancer, and visualize the obvious differences in your stance, intent, and touching objectives compared to the previous two exercises.

### ■  MENTAL EXERCISE 4  ■

Another good mental exercise is to perform a 10-minute seated tune-up either blindfolded or with your eyes closed throughout the entire 10 minutes. This enables you to focus on the function of your hands as vehicles of communication. These exercises also enhance your versatility in personalizing Performance Massage to the recipient.

## Preparing Your Hands

Hands are the primary vehicle for nonverbal communication. Hands can do many things—strike a blow, make a fist, ask for spare change, establish a boundary, offer encouragement, provide relief, offer comfort, and establish our basic connection with others. Touch is our first and primary sense, and the hands are the special instruments of touch.

Care and use of the hands are all-important when providing massage. You will find it helpful not to wear rings, watches, or other jewelry when massaging. Wash your hands before and after every session, and keep your fingernails short enough that they do not scratch or irritate the skin.

Keep your hands warm and dry prior to massaging. You may wish to warm them under hot water, particularly if the recipient is chilled or the room temperature is not optimally warm (usually around 72°F, or 22°C).

When you perform massage, your hands impart the nonverbal intent of your session. Seldom are the hands required to assume highly stressful positions during massage. Some practicing therapists do, however, develop arthritis in the fingers and wrists and tendinitis in the thumbs. Carpal tunnel syndrome can also develop if the wrist is excessively hyperextended while applying pressure. To avoid these problems, keep your hands relaxed and maintain a straight line of energy flow through the shoulders, elbows, wrists, and hands. Failure to do this may unnecessarily stress the joints of the thumb, fingers, or wrist. If you do develop pain, immediately stop performing the given techniques and utilize other strokes that feel comfortable.

By exercising and strengthening your hands, you will find it much easier to keep proper alignment. Hand exercises include squeezing a hand grip, performing modified push-ups on the fingertips, and simple range of motion movements that spread the fingers and then squeeze them together. Many gyms and health clubs have wrist-rolling and forearm-strengthening machines that can also develop the flexors and extensors of the hand. However, if you are doing massage on an occasional basis, you will probably not develop any overuse stresses or strains.

If your hands, and particularly your thumbs, are hypermobile (loose-jointed), be especially careful when you apply the cross-fiber friction stroke. As you can see from the following illustrations, if your thumbs are adequately supported by your fingers, and your alignment stays straight, you can employ maximal pressure without straining your joints. However, if your thumbs tend to collapse as shown in the second picture, this will unduly stress the joints and the surrounding connective tissue. My suggestion would be to use the splinted-finger approach as discussed on page 83 when you apply cross-fiber friction. This is both appropriately specific and more user-friendly to the practitioner.

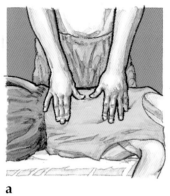 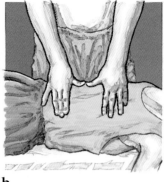

**Keep your thumbs supported by your fingers (a) to use maximal pressure without straining your joints. Collapsing your thumbs (b) stresses your joints.**

a                               b

## Acquiring the Basic Skills

In addition to readying yourself mentally and preparing your hands for massage, you will also need to acquire a few basic skills that are important no matter which technique you're using. You will need to know the correct way to apply leverage, breathe, develop a sense of touch, sense tension, find trigger points, and personalize the massage.

### Leverage and Leaning

An essential concept in Performance Massage is the appropriate use of body weight and proper biomechanics. This means using your weight and not your strength to apply pressure. If you use only the strength of your arms, hands, and shoulders, you will tire quickly, and the person you are massaging will sense your own physical strain and exertion.

It is important to relax your arms and hands completely and move your body into a lunge position, where your front foot is pointing in the direction of your force (similar to the stance of a boxer) and your rear foot is anchored, in order that you may shift your body weight back and forth as pressure requires.

It is essential that you learn how to extend your arms and use your leverage when applying Performance Massage. This will transmit a sense of touch that is relaxing and beneficial rather than strained and tense.

These are the key points in utilizing your body:

- Keep your knees bent, and feel the weight of your body shift as you lean back and forth.
- Point your front foot in the direction of your technique.

- Raise the heel of your rear foot to apply additional leverage, transmitting body weight, not strength, onto your partner.
- Keep your arms and hands relaxed.
- Keep your arms in extension with very little bending at the elbows.

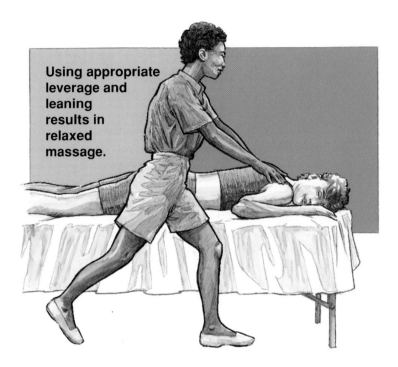

**Using appropriate leverage and leaning results in relaxed massage.**

If possible, watch yourself in a mirror as you lean, shift, apply pressure, change directions, and integrate your strokes. This can greatly assist you in forming a tableside position that is efficient and nonfatiguing. Also be sure to keep your chin tucked and your head in proper alignment to conclude a structurally stable approach. Massage requires not great strength but rather a knowledge and awareness of body mechanics.

If you keep your body relaxed, both you and your partner will enjoy an effective and therapeutic session.

## Breathing!

A common mistake of many massage therapists and bodyworkers is holding the breath when applying specific or deep techniques. This is counterproductive, because your body begins to tighten and strain, losing the graceful and intuitive approach to the recipient.

Consciously focus on your breathing while applying Performance Massage. Occasionally take a deep "diaphragmatic breath" and feel the movement in your trunk and throughout your rib cage. This three-dimensional breathing will offer both you and your partner an opportunity to "hook up" to each other's internal rhythms and pacings.

You will find that, at the completion of your session, you will be less fatigued, have better endurance, and feel a sense of relaxation. Breathing is an essential component of life. By making this a priority in your massage, you can greatly enhance its therapeutic effects.

## Developing a Sense of Touch

Developing a sense of touch requires intuition, or "sixth sense." Intuition includes the unspoken nuances of our hands-on session. To be intuitive means to "listen" to our senses, especially our hands, our sense of touch, to discover what part of the body might be sore or injured. We also allow the hunches and guesses of the exploratory process to enter into our massage approach.

Dogs are by nature highly intuitive and in some cultures are major symbols of the intuitive process. Dogs are often alert to new possibilities, new adventures, new horizons. They can "sniff out" the right direction and have great trust in the power of instinct. Developing the sixth sense of the canny canine will foster hand movements that "sniff out" trigger points and tender spots. An intuitive touch will prevent your massage from becoming routine or mechanical. You can set the stage for development of creative and intuitive touch by staying relaxed, quiet, and "in touch" with the nonverbal communication between you and the recipient. It may include a deep sigh, a quiet smile, a letting go of tension, or a subtle drowsiness. As you develop an exploratory and highly sensitive sense of touch, you will note that this component is as essential as any technical skill in providing quality hands-on care.

I would also suggest that you consider studying the major muscles of the body and acquaint yourself with the basics of surface anatomy (see Appendix B). This knowledge will anchor the foundation required for safe and specific massage therapy. Knowledge and creativity are not mutually exclusive traits, but rather are essential components of "touch literacy."

***Guidelines to Foster an Educated Touch.***    Totally relax during the massage and consciously let go of any tension, stress, or negative thoughts you may be carrying. This sets the stage for a positive hook-up between you and the athlete.

Breathe! Inhale through your nose slowly to the count of 6, and then gently exhale through your mouth to the same count. Notice the dry coolness of the air as it enters the nose and its moist warmth while it is being expelled through the mouth. Note the three-dimensional aspect of your breathing. Feel your lungs and diaphragm move, rib cage expand, and soft tissues relax as your breathing becomes deeper and fuller.

Vary the tempo of your massage. You can greatly enhance your touch skills by using soft background music, particularly classical jazz, which provides a beat, a harmony, and an improvisational theme. While practicing your massage skills, try slowing down and speeding up your tempo throughout the session to create a specific effect on the muscles. How you vary the tempo, pressure, and integration of your massage often determines your overall success.

Experiment with your pressure. Remember that most areas of the body contain several layers of muscle tissue separated by layers of fascia. Some parts of the body, such as the upper back and feet, have four layers of muscle. By experimenting with your force, you can feel a sense of melting, or release, in superficial tissues as you gently, yet firmly, engage the deeper holding patterns—configurations that soft tissues assume as a result of stress or tension. Keep in mind that "working deep is not working hard." It is essential to use leverage and leaning (and not arm strength) when giving deep massage. This is especially true when working with heavyweight wrestlers, shot-putters, and weight lifters.

Visualization can enhance the therapeutic effectiveness of your touch. I often visualize the veins and arteries and musculature as being congested in the same way that piping of a sink or a drain becomes clogged. As you apply compression and appropriate pressure, imagine how a fresh supply of oxygenated blood is decongesting the physical structure. As the skin becomes more pliable and warmer and assumes a reddish hue, I realize that I have initiated a circulatory flush. Those images correspond with my hands-on techniques creating optimal results.

***Touch as Service.***    Touch is a component of service. By providing service in a clear, uncomplicated, and caring fashion, you can't help but convey feelings of safety, trust, and pleasure. Touch is a marvelous tool among all living creatures in establishing this connection. Your success in developing a sense of touch only adds to your ability to generate positive physical and psychological effects.

The recipient of your massage is somebody special! Any time you are providing hands-on therapy in the form of massage, the technique, sequence, and anything you have read in this or any other book is secondary to the person receiving the massage. Make that person your top priority, and allow your knowledge and creativity to serve her or his unique physiological condition. Remember that this condition, particularly among physically active people, can change dramatically day to day, depending on recent training, workouts, levels of exhaustion, and day-to-day well-being. There is a fine line between being properly trained and being overtrained. By keying in on the individual needs and physical symptoms of your partner, you can enhance his or her self-esteem through your massage session.

## Sensing Tension

When giving massage, you will be able to intuit much of your partner's tension through the various sensations you obtain through your hands and fingers. However, there are other nonverbal ways in which the location of tension can be communicated. Often you will experience a reflexive tightening or holding if you get to an area of constriction or soreness. Additionally, your partner may make a face, such as a grimace, that indicates that you may be going too deep or that the area is markedly sore. You will occasionally notice a tightening of the jaw and the facial muscles or a mask-like expression on the face. This is simply your partner's method of indicating an area of tension, or of "holding on."

Be respectful and massage only within the limits of your partner's comfort zone. This shows respect and an ability to work cooperatively, as opposed to doing a generic massage.

Often you will notice that areas of muscle tightness appear white, clammy, or cold to the touch. This is a result of soft-tissue restrictions causing ischemia, which occurs when knotted muscles cut off the supply of oxygen-rich blood. Pain will increase in these areas, because the muscle cannot take in oxygen and cannot wash away the toxic buildup of lactic acid and other waste products.

Develop your intuition. Your skills in performing Performance Massage will develop rapidly.

Fully surrendering to and enjoying a therapeutic massage can be one of life's most fundamental and profound pleasures. This just might be the beginning of an ongoing therapeutic adventure!

## Finding Trigger Points

Trigger points are those hypersensitive, tiny areas within muscle fibers that are tender to the touch and often send, or refer, pain to other parts of the body. When performance intensity outweighs the body's ability to withstand physical stress, the muscles will reflexively tighten, and trigger points can develop. Sometimes these are the source of ropiness or tautness within the fibers or feel like a nodule or taut band.

In the course of providing Performance Massage, you will be assessing the skin through a layer of clothing in search of these exquisitely tender points. Although trigger points can occur in any of the body's 600 or so muscles, they are particularly common in the upper back, neck, and low back areas. The purpose in finding these tender spots is to neutralize the pain referral that accompanies them and help bring about the restoration of maximal muscle functioning.

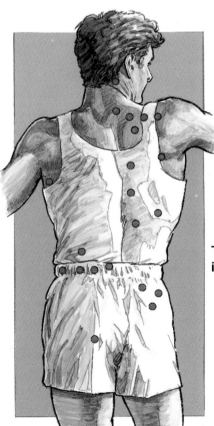

**Trigger points are common in the back and neck.**

There are several methods of seeking out trigger point locations, including compression and the pincer technique, which are described fully in chapter 5. You can also notice if the massage recipient performs spontaneous stretching movements for relief in an area that is short or restricted. Additionally, when addressed with direct pressure, the recipient may exhibit a twitch response, or a jump sign. This is an involuntary twitch in reaction to the excessive neurological activity within the point itself. Through an awareness of the stresses typical of a particular sport or workout regimen, you can often go directly to the muscles that are usually overloaded and zero in on these sensitive pain sites. Take care not to gouge or poke at these tender spots.

Mapping the body for trigger points involves being a good detective on your part. Listen to the body. Note any irregularities, and ask for specific feedback as you probe, knead, and compress the musculature for these "zingers." This assessment technique will greatly enhance your ability to restore the muscle to normal functioning and relieve pain. I often instruct those I massage to breathe into the tenderness as direct pressure is being applied, to facilitate a release or letting-go of the trigger point. This procedure is extremely effective for reducing pain and restoring the recipient to optimal physical functioning.

If much of your massage session involves neutralizing these points, the massage recipient will benefit from taking a warm shower afterward and then performing some slow, easy stretching movements. By doing this, she or he can experience not only a reduction of muscle irritation, but a softening and freeing of the involved tissues. This alone can provide the physical and psychological edge conducive to doing any activity to one's fullest potential.

The muscle diagram in Appendix B shows the location of some of the most common trigger points in active people. However, this is merely presented as a guideline. By developing your palpatory skills and spending time on rolling, broadening, and applying direct pressure to the tissues, you can become quite skillful at searching out trigger points. Remember, your fingers are acting as sensors as you gently and cooperatively unravel and loosen the overworked tissues. Be certain that your objectives are coordinated with a vigilant sensitivity and a cooperative relationship with the person on the table. Employing too much pressure too soon or having the recipient reflexively tighten is counterproductive to the neutralization of these trigger points.

## Personalizing the Massage

Over the years I have massaged dancers, amputees, professional wrestlers, marathon champions, special-needs athletes in wheelchairs, martial arts practitioners, competitive body builders, grandmothers, drug-exposed infants, yoga instructors, the drummer for the Beatles, notorious gangsters, world-class sprinters, and thousands upon thousands of individuals hoping to feel better and improve their physical fitness. Needless to say, each one of these persons received a different massage!

My point is that the entire content and all of the techniques of massage are specifically geared to the individual needs and physical condition of the person receiving it. Nothing is more important than the person on the table. The rate, rhythm, duration, techniques employed, areas given special attention, and tempo all depend upon the individual. This is why it is so important that you develop the sense-of-touch skills discussed on page 40. Massage is sometimes called a psychophysical art. Like music, it has mathematical, creative, structural, and improvisational qualities. The most successful massage practitioners are those who routinely employ this creative improvisational approach to provide the best possible comfort, relief, and total-body experience for the person on the table.

If you routinely follow a generic or mechanized sequence as outlined in so many massage books, you will soon find your sessions becoming dull and limited in their therapeutic potency. Because each person is different, you will need to attune yourself to the muscle texture, the overall body tension, the desired effect of the session, and the optimal impact zone (the ideal receptivity range) of every individual. I can attest that this varies greatly from person to person.

Varying rhythm is another way of personalizing the massage. Rhythm and tempo indicate the speed at which you integrate breathing, movement, and other aspects of techniques. For example, if your partner is tense and nervous, you may wish to establish a slow rhythm to counter this. You will find that this has a relaxing impact and that usually within a few minutes your partner's breath will be deeper, the muscles more elastic, and your partner will be more receptive.

If, however, your partner is lethargic, you may wish to quicken your rhythm. This will induce circulatory stimulation and the release of trapped energy. Your partner will inevitably feel more energetic and alert.

You may wish to alternate your rhythm by beginning your massage with a slow, steady application of strokes. Gradually you can increase the tempo and rhythm by applying your sequence more briskly. If your partner seems receptive to this, continue in this fashion for a few minutes. Then, gradually begin to slow down and work deeper and more thoroughly on areas of stress and holding. This is particularly effective on the back, allowing you to pay special attention to tender spots and tight muscles.

Be certain that your transitions are not jerky or disconnected, because this makes your movements seem careless. Do not suddenly make or break contact, as this can provide a slight shock to the muscle and nervous systems.

Expertise in rhythm and tempo comes only through practicing speed and the transition from one technique to another. It is very effective to close your eyes occasionally and become conscious of the speed of your sequence. By varying the rhythm and tempo, you can become more intuitive and far more receptive to your partner's holding patterns and body armoring.

## Preparing the Recipient

In addition to preparing yourself mentally and acquiring the basic skills for effective massage sessions, it's important to prepare each individual to receive a massage. You should set some ground rules for communicating during the session and make sure the recipient understands how to position him- or herself on the table.

### Communication During Performance Massage

Some individuals will talk compulsively, which can stress the jaw, throat, and neck. Often this masks discomfort or stress. Be conscious of this, and set the stage for nonverbal communication.

Explain that talking during a massage is counterproductive to the communication that you are establishing with your hands. If you stay focused with your head, heart, and hands, there seldom will be a need for verbal dialogue, except for an occasional check to see how the pressure or the massage is going. Use silence to increase intuition and relaxation, and encourage the recipient to consider massage time as "prime time." Soft music can reduce the awkwardness that may occur at first.

If an individual does talk and it seems to add to the encounter, feel free to respond, but try to avoid controversial issues such as religion, politics, and finances. By letting your partner initiate the conversation, you will be respecting her or his right to personalize the experience. If talking becomes excessive, however, gently suggest that it may be a good idea to focus on breathing and to make mental notes as to where tension or stress is experienced. Also, it is a good idea to have your partner focus on a pleasant thought, location, or experience in order to enhance receptivity. Techniques that enhance body/mind interaction can facilitate a lengthening and letting-go of muscle restriction.

Begin your treatment by clearly informing your partner about what to expect, how long the session will last, and his or her responsibility in the session to give you feedback about pressure and tempo. Tell your partner to communicate what feels especially good. In this setting, you will find the need to talk diminished, and the conversation that does occur will only improve your massage.

## Positioning on the Table

There are three positions that the recipient will assume on the massage table while you are giving a Performance Massage.

**Supine.**   The first of these positions is the supine, or face up, position. Make certain that your partner is comfortable on the table, and, if requested, place a small pillow under her or his neck to support the head. Ideally, the pillow should be no more than 2 inches thick.

It is also sometimes helpful to place rolled-up towels or additional pillows under your partner's knees to allow the legs to relax in the position of maximum comfort.

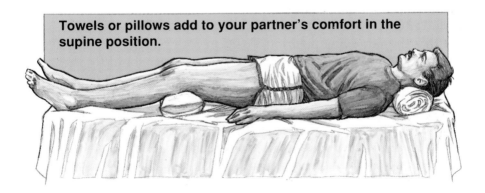

**Towels or pillows add to your partner's comfort in the supine position.**

***Prone.***    Many of your Performance Massage techniques will be used while your partner is in the prone, or face down, position. Once again make sure that your partner is comfortable on the table, and, if warranted, place a rolled-up towel or a pillow under the ankles or have your partner hang his or her feet off the end of the table. This will keep the feet muscles from cramping, which may occur if the feet are pressed into the surface. The recipient may be more comfortable with a small pillow or folded towel under the head or chest, turning the head to whatever side is comfortable. However, have your partner turn the head to the opposite side several times while in the prone position to avoid any stiffening in the neck muscles. The arms can be placed alongside the head in a bent position with the hands resting on either side of the head, or allow the arms to hang off the side of the table if that is more comfortable.

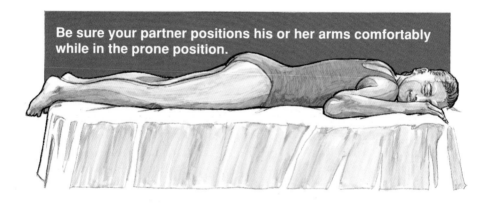

Be sure your partner positions his or her arms comfortably while in the prone position.

***Side-Lying***    The third position your partner will be in while you work is the side-lying position. Position your partner so that there is a straight line (as illustrated) through the ear, shoulder, hip, extended knee, and ankle. The upper leg is to be flexed at the hip and at the knee so that there is a straight line through the waistline and the flexed knee. This creates an inverted figure-four position.

When your partner is in the side-lying position, a pillow under the head and a rolled-up towel or a small pillow under the flexed knee can enhance relaxation and comfort.

For best results, see to it that your partner is always comfortable on the table and that he or she feels a sense of relaxation or "sinking in to the surface." Have your partner focus on his or her breathing, close the eyes, and remember to turn or change positions on the table in a slow and deliberate manner. Remember, this is downtime for all involved.

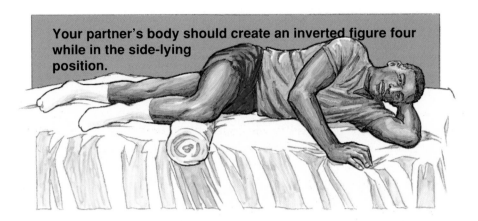

Your partner's body should create an inverted figure four while in the side-lying position.

## Receiving a Massage

If you are learning Performance Massage with a training partner as I suggested in the introduction, there will be times when you are the recipient of a massage. You may need a bit of preparation for this.

For many people, this is a surprising topic. Countless individuals are now enjoying the pleasure and relaxation of ongoing massage experiences and find little difficulty in relaxing, letting go, or fully appreciating this highly effective art form. However, no two people are alike, and depending on your past touch history, you may find the following recommendations helpful in receiving the many beneficial and therapeutic effects of Performance Massage.

If you feel modest or awkward about being touched, convey this to your partner so that there is an understanding at the very beginning of the session that you as the recipient are in control of the session. This means that if you want less pressure applied or you do not want to be given a certain technique that you find unpleasant or you simply choose to conclude the treatment at any given point, these wishes will be respected. Once you realize that your personal boundaries are being respected, you can more fully relax and submit to the many pleasurable sensations of therapeutic massage.

As a general rule, offer spontaneous feedback as the session is progressing. This gives you the opportunity to direct your partner's efforts in accordance with your receptivity. You will find it helpful, however, to speak only when necessary and to allow for the fact that this is your time—and your opportunity to go inward into a deep state of relaxation. Not surprisingly, you may experience a softening or letting-go of mental and emotional stress, anxiety, and tension as the body begins to unwind and relax.

Inhaling slowly and deeply through the nose and exhaling through the mouth can also enhance the therapeutic value of your massage and make it easier to let go of body fatigue. Make certain that you are comfortable while on the table, and don't feel that you need to "cooperate" with your partner by moving, lifting, or assisting in the session. Let your partner perform the manipulations and strokes. Allow yourself to become passive and receptive to the massage experience.

If these are new sensations for you, massage can be an especially delightful experience. Consider the session a reward for the commitment you have shown to achieving success and physical fitness.

During the massage, see if you can fully experience some of the beneficial effects of the session. Allow yourself to feel the fluids moving in your body's extremities. Notice the feeling of weightlessness as a limb is lifted and stretched. Visualize the increased pliability and suppleness of the skin as it responds to the squeezing and rolling techniques. Notice the warm, glowing feeling as blood circulation is increased. Another sensation I enjoy is the feeling of decongestion or unwinding within the muscles that I often overwork. See if you can fully experience the nerve endings becoming calm and any deep aches leaving your body. Your self-esteem can also be enhanced if you consciously give yourself permission to enjoy to the fullest possible extent the massage experience. Remember, this is one of the few health habits that not only is good for you, but feels good. Therapeutic massage has no calories, white sugar, cholesterol, or artificial substances, but it may still have addictive side effects!

## General Guidelines
## for Practicing Performance Massage

I've given you a lot of information in this chapter, but you needn't feel overwhelmed. You'll learn best by practicing. There is no substitute for performing the techniques on a regular basis, however awkward you may feel at first. You may be surprised at how quickly your confidence develops and how you internalize not only the technique sequences but your own variations on Performance Massage.

Allow yourself some initial awkwardness. You may find that the intimacy of touch is problematic for you or your training partner. You may also feel unskilled at practicing this nonverbal yet powerful form of communication. A sense of humor goes a long way toward easing the tension you may feel. An honest exchange of feedback can also give you the necessary information for developing Performance Massage skills. Have a clear understanding with your partner that if any components of your hands-on session don't feel right, it is OK to exchange information and feedback without any sense of blaming. This sets the stage for productive communication that enhances your learning process.

Stay focused on the intent and objectives of your session. By getting in touch with this "softer side" of yourself, you can set aside judgmental or overly critical self-assessments. Keep in mind that touch is as natural as fresh air, food, and proper rest for growth and development of the human species. Occasionally give the type of session that you yourself would experience as wonderful. On a subconscious level many professionals often master the very style and approach that they themselves are most receptive to.

While giving a massage, it is OK to acknowledge that you feel awkward or uncomfortable or that you are self-conscious. You can diffuse any escalating negative feelings by consciously relaxing and focusing on your sense of service. You are learning a pleasurable and effective art form.

Again, you will find it helpful to give massage in a room with a mirror. This will enable you to assess and become more fully conscious of your own holding patterns or areas of postural stress. It took me several years before I fully understood the essence of postural alignment. Get comfortable!

Learning any new skill takes time and patience. My experience is that Performance Massage is one of the easiest approaches to learn, because it requires only a fundamental grasp of basic hand positions and also encourages the intuition, blending, sensitivity, and integration that is unique to activity refinement. Like any peak performance, your coordination, grace, and follow-through will soon become effortless and personally expressive. This sets the stage for hands-on therapy that is mutually fulfilling, highly therapeutic, and a pleasure to give and receive.

# Chapter 5

# Techniques of Performance Massage

nowing something about musical composition does not make one a musician. Understanding sport biomechanics does not automatically make one a good athlete. Nor does a rational, left-brain understanding of massage techniques guarantee a gifted session. There must be a balance between understanding and intuition in the practice and mastery of this psychophysical art.

My descriptions of Performance Massage strokes will teach you hand positioning, which body parts each technique benefits, and other application specifics. But at the same time I encourage you to experiment with the subtleties of massage, allowing your hands to become sensors, feeling and probing for areas of restriction or tenderness. Try to keep a balance between learning the form and applying it intuitively. The dynamism between these two approaches encourages necessary skill development and improvisational proficiency.

## Getting Started

Start with the beginning sequence of strokes on page 55 to become familiar both with the techniques themselves and with their gradual progression from general to specific. Chart your progress and seek feedback from your partner as you begin learning these hands-on skills. Remember, it is natural to feel awkward or clumsy or self-conscious at first, because our culture is not primarily a touching one. As you develop skills and receive positive responses from your partner, you will boost your self-confidence and your influence on your partner's athletic or artistic performance. Also remember that all of the techniques and approaches in this book are designed to serve the physical and mental condition of the person on the table. Be responsive to any feedback from your partner, and try to gauge your efforts toward enhancing your partner's wellness and relaxation.

As you're learning, read the description of the technique to your partner. Study the accompanying photograph, and then apply the stroke to your partner. Using this method, you can conceptualize the stroke, visualize the application as portrayed in the picture, and then perform the technique with immediate feedback to fine-tune your applications. I have found that this method creates a stress-free environment in which to learn to develop sound two-way communication between partners.

Perhaps most important in getting started is to devote sufficient time to practicing the strokes and getting feedback. Although Performance Massage is normally done in a 20-minute sequence, it will take you several hours of practice, feedback, and self-correction for a smooth session to emerge. Be patient, allow for the learning time you need, and, above all, take pride in the powerful therapeutic skill that you are learning.

Both Performance Massage and exercise have the goal of keeping muscles and circulatory fluids relaxed, healthy, and in optimal condition. With this goal in mind, let's begin applying the techniques of Performance Massage.

# *Energy Moves*
## *Stretch Tissues and Unwind Muscles*

Energy moves are used to loosen and stretch connective tissue, to increase circulation, and unwind tight muscles. These techniques, including rocking, shaking, and vibration, help you to familiarize your sense of touch to the recipient's body and prepare the tissues for deeper work. Energy moves should be applied at a relatively brisk pace; they will stimulate and energize.

# *Rocking*

Rocking is a good way to start the session. Rhythmic rocking relaxes the individual while introducing gentle motion to the body. It is primarily used with the recipient in the prone position.

Place your hands on the back with your fingertips pointing away from you. Start by exerting a forward pressure with the heels of your hands, moving the body slightly away from you. Follow this with a pulling motion with your fingertips to return the body to its original position.

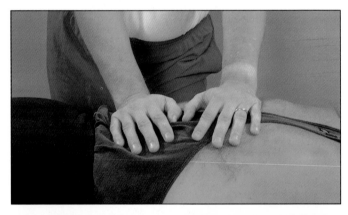

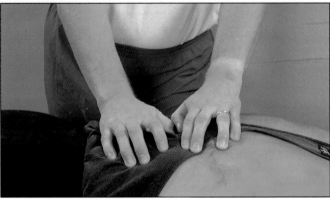

Push with the heels, pull with the fingertips.

By slightly changing the position of your hands as you start a gentle back-and-forth movement, you will become familiar with the contours of the body. Be sensitive to the body's own natural rhythm, and keep the pace of your rocking in harmony with it.

As you progress through the following variations, you will feel the segments of the body moving independently.

## *Variation 1:   Sacrum/Back*

Rock the lower back with one hand placed directly above the sacrum while stabilizing the mid-back area with the other hand.

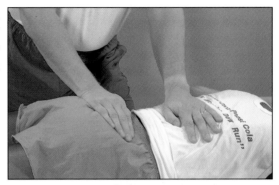

Rock the sacrum
while stabilizing the mid-back.

## *Variation 2:   Hamstrings/Back*

Rock the posterior thighs with one hand placed directly on the hamstrings while exerting a slight pressure on the lower back with the other hand.

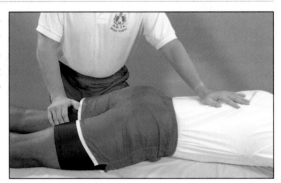

Rock the hamstrings
while stabilizing the low back.

## *Variation 3:   Sacral Stretching*

Exert a slight downward pull on the sacrum while rocking it with one hand, and a slight upward compression on each side of the spine with the other hand.

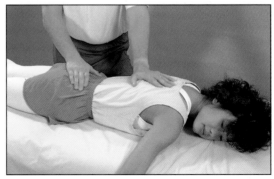

Apply downward pressure on the sacrum
while stabilizing the mid-back.

# *Shaking*

Shaking the arms and legs while exerting a gentle traction will help the recipient "let go." As the connective tissue is stretched, your partner will feel a sense of weightlessness in the limbs, which will help him or her relax.

To shake the legs, stand at the foot of the table, wrap the palm of your hand around the top of the foot while stabilizing the heel with your other hand. This grip will enable you to mobilize the leg without putting any pressure on the ankle.

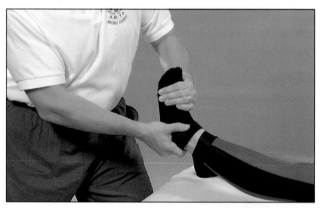

Carefully hold the foot and ankle while applying traction to the limb.

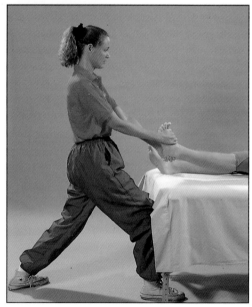

While maintaining this grip, you can perform a *limb pull* by exerting a gentle traction on the leg, bending your knees, and leaning slightly backward. Combine the leg pull with a light shaking or bouncing, keeping in mind that the motion should come from the hip and not just the lower leg.

Bend your knees and lean backward to stretch the leg.

To shake the arms, stand at the side of the table, grasp the hand by placing both of your thumbs on the top of the hand and your fingers on the palm of the hand as pictured. Keep your grip well below the wrist so that the hand will not flop when you shake the arm.

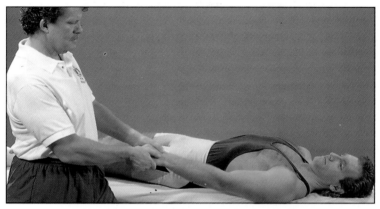

Stabilize your partner's hand during shaking.

As with the leg, perform a limb pull on the arm by exerting a gentle traction, bending your knees, and leaning slightly backward. Change your position slightly as you shake or bounce the arm to get mobility in the shoulder joint.

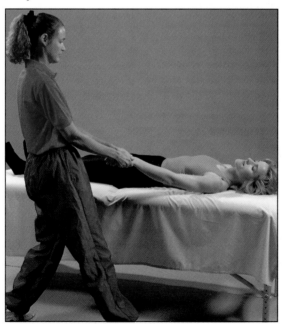

Leaning back, apply sustained pressure to the joints of the arm.

# Vibration

Vibration loosens the connective tissues, stimulates nerve endings, and encourages deeper lymphatic and venous circulation. Add a slight trembling motion to your hands and arms as you move them over the body. This rapid shaking imparts a tremulous impact, causing that body part to vibrate. As the tissues unwind, you can progress from superficial to deep by applying more pressure.

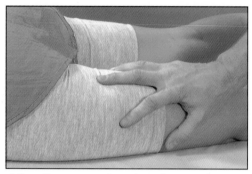

Rapidly vibrate your hands to loosen the tissues.

Vibration can be used to complement other techniques and can be applied in any direction (e.g., toward you, away from you). You can move your hand along the body as you apply vibration, or you can sink in and work in one spot for a while.

The recipient will feel the sensation of vibration in different ways as you shift the pressure from the palm of your hand to the fingertips. Use both hands, or use one hand while stabilizing with the other.

## Variation :   Bear Claw

Spread your fingers like bear claws and exert pressure with your fingertips as you apply vibration. The tremulous effect will be imparted through each of your fingers, causing that body part to gently loosen.

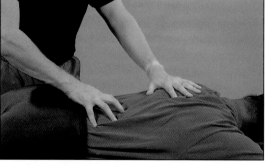

Spread your fingers and apply fingertip vibration.

# *Abdominal Sandwich*

Stand perpendicular to your partner who is lying supine on the table. Place one hand under the lumbar curve of the lower back just above the sacrum and your other hand on the lower abdominal muscles just below the navel. Ask your partner to raise your top hand by slowly breathing into it. This technique allows for a three-dimensional diaphragmatic breath, which is relaxing and calming before exertion.

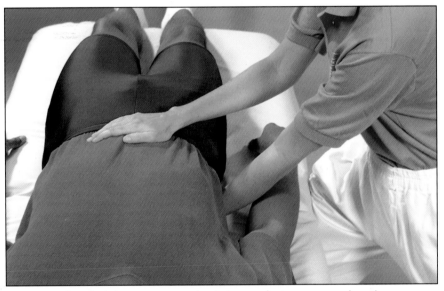

Sandwich your partner's abdomen between your hands
as he or she raises your hand by breathing deeply.

# Muscle Flushing
## Decongest and Oxygenate Muscles

Muscle flushing techniques are designed to wring, roll, squeeze, decongest, and flush metabolic wastes and toxins from the musculature. This condition, called ischemia, is followed by a hyperemia that bathes the tissues in a fresh supply of oxygenated blood and nutrients.

As you knead the tissues, your fingers will provide you with clues to the condition of the musculature. You will be able to determine muscle tone, temperature, tension, and tenderness. (Areas that have decreased circulation will feel cold; areas that are inflamed or that have increased circulation will feel hot.)

In addition to their stimulating effect on the circulatory system, muscle flushing techniques increase tissue pliability.

# *Kneading*

Kneading is a great way to get blood into the tissues before a workout and metabolites out of the muscles after a workout. You can markedly decrease the recovery time after a strenuous workout by manually pumping lactic acid and other metabolites out of the muscles. Kneading the tissues will actively stimulate the flow of blood and lymph, which can decrease muscle soreness caused by the accumulation of lactic acid.

Grasp the muscle and hold it between the thumb and fingers of one or both hands. Make sure that you are engaging the muscle and not just the skin. Squeeze, lift, and stretch the tissue by alternately grasping and releasing segments of the musculature.

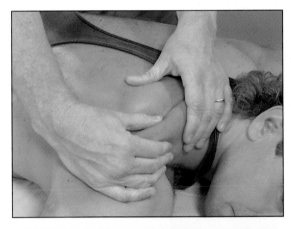

Kneading should be done deeply enough to lift the musculature away from the underlying bones and to free and separate the muscle fibers. Be sensitive as you progress from superficial to deep levels. Your partner may already have some muscle soreness, especially after a heavy workout.

Take time to work thoroughly around the shoulder, upper arm, back, and gluteals. Tailor the session to the needs of the individual: Dancers need a lot of work on the thigh and calf muscles, swimmers need work on the pectoral area.

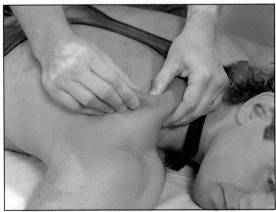

Knead the muscle by alternately grasping and releasing the tissues.

# *Skin Rolling*

Skin needs exercise too! Skin rolling increases the skin's pliability and circulation.

Skin rolling is great for the skin and the superficial muscles of the lower back. In addition to flushing the area with oxygenated blood and nutrients, it allows the muscles greater freedom of movement by stretching the adjacent connective tissues.

Skin rolling is done in a progressive manner over the surface of the back by picking up successive segments of skin between the fingers and thumbs while moving smoothly in one direction. Allow slack to develop in the skin by placing your four fingers one or two inches away from your thumb. Walk your fingers in any direction with the thumbs gliding behind. This will allow the slackened tissue to roll between your thumbs and fingers.

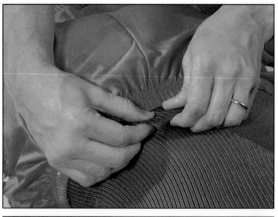

As you work thoroughly over the lower back, you should be able to feel temperature variations (if any) on the surface of the skin. (Areas that have decreased circulation will feel cold; areas that are inflamed or that have increased circulation will feel hot.)

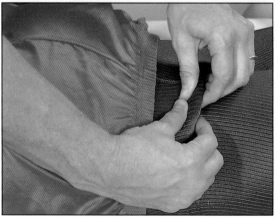

Roll the slackened tissue
between your thumbs and fingers.

# *Fascial Pickup*

A great tension reliever, fascial pickup lets the muscles move freely by loosening the superficial fascia.

Standing alongside the table, reach across your partner to the opposite side and place your hands on the muscles of the back. Grasp a fold of skin between the fingertips and heels of your hands. Lift the tissue upward, apply a gentle shake, and release.

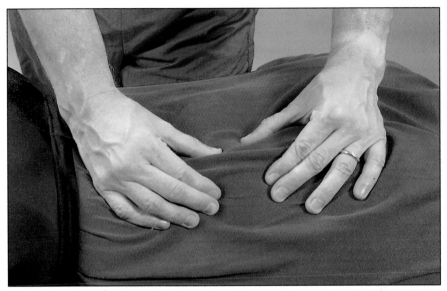

Gently shake the tissue as you grasp and lift.

Take time to work thoroughly over the entire surface of the back.

# *Pincer Grip*

A highly specific access technique for trouble spots, the pincer grip lets you apply pressure to a muscle from opposite directions. Applying sustained pressure is a good way to get a contracted muscle to release.

Grasp the muscle with the thumb, the index finger, and perhaps the middle finger. Maintain a steady pressure, gently shake the tissue, then release.

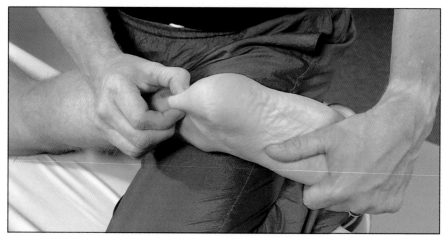

Apply a pincer grip to the Achilles tendon.

The muscles in the back of the neck, the trapezius, and the Achilles tendon respond well to this technique.

# *Rotary Thumb Probe*

Use the rotary thumb probe to restore elasticity and suppleness to muscles and to neutralize areas of muscle soreness in athletes suffering from chronic back pain. This technique is both general and specific in that it lets you warm the tissues with the broad application of your hand while locating and neutralizing areas of muscle soreness with your thumb. This technique allows you to work very deeply with your thumb because of the "distraction" of grasping the adjacent tissue. As your hand provides a general toning to the musculature, your thumb will neutralize muscle soreness by direct fiber spreading.

Soft-tissue twisting movements are effective in releasing adhesions, which are caused by microtrauma or injury and interfere with muscle contraction. The twisting thumb compression applied in the rotary thumb probe helps muscles maintain a supple texture by separating and stretching the fibers and thereby releasing any adhesions.

Place one hand on the muscle, making firm contact with the thumb and fingers. As you work the tissue by grasping portions of muscle with one hand, use the thumb of your other hand to apply a twisting compression within the angle formed by your thumb and index finger.

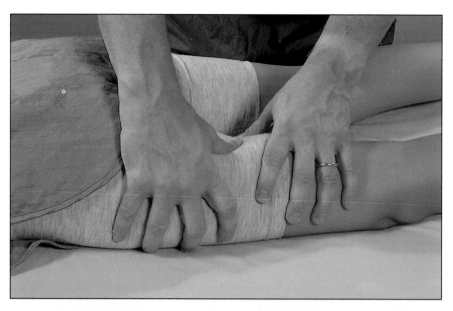

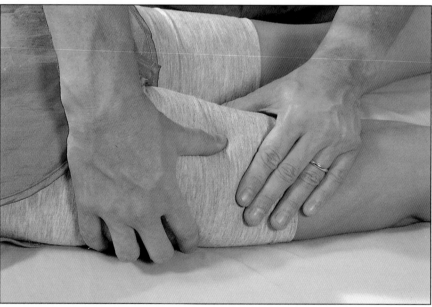

Press your thumb into the slackened area created by your other hand.

This technique allows you to work very deeply with your thumb, because of the distraction of grasping the adjacent tissue. As your hand provides a general toning to the musculature, your thumb will probe deeper structures.

Work thoroughly over the back, gluteals, and hamstrings.

# *Heel Squeeze*

The heel squeeze is great for applying a two-sided compression to large muscles.

As in the pincer grip, squeezing with the heel of your hand lets you apply pressure to a muscle from opposite directions. However, because you use the heels of both hands rather than the thumb and one or two fingers, you can engage a larger muscle area.

Intertwine the fingers of both hands and place the heels on each side of the muscle. Keep your hands in line with your forearms so you do not stress your wrists. Grasp the middle, or belly, of the muscle between the heels of your hands, and squeeze to compress the tissues.

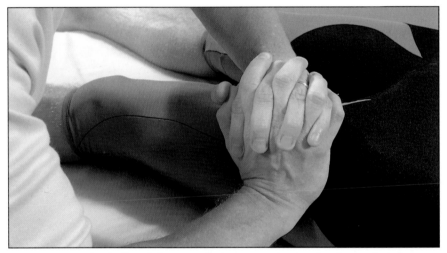

Squeeze the belly of the muscle between the heels of your hands.

Work the entire length of the leg, front and back, to compress the hamstrings, quadriceps, calf muscles, and iliotibial band. Avoid the area directly behind the knee.

# Pressure Techniques
## Spread Muscle Fibers
## and Nourish Muscles

Pressure techniques are most effective when you use your body weight and leverage to deliver direct pressure to the natural contours of the musculature. Rhythmic compression spreads the muscle fibers, enhancing their ability to contract and relax as well as bringing more nutrients and oxygen to the muscles.

# *Stretch and Twist Compression*

Stretch and twist compression is a powerful technique that lengthens and unwinds tight musculature. The person who is tense or whose muscles are tightly contracted will benefit greatly from stretch and twist compression. The application of pressure in this technique is accompanied by a gentle traction to create space between your hands, lengthening the superficial fascia and underlying musculature.

To allow you to deliver enough pressure to the musculature, the table should be low enough that you can place your hands on the muscles with your arms fully extended and your knees slightly bent. This will enable you to use your body's leverage to deliver appropriate pressure while changing positions as you move around the body.

*Note.* Keep your elbows slightly bent as you compress the tissues—do not absorb the impact by excessively bending your elbows.

Mold your hand to the contours of the musculature as you apply pressure using the heel of your hand, following this with a slight twist of the whole arm. Alternate your hands while reinforcing the compression of each hand with the leverage of your body. You can exert a gentle traction at the same time by spreading your hands slightly away from each other as you compress the tissues.

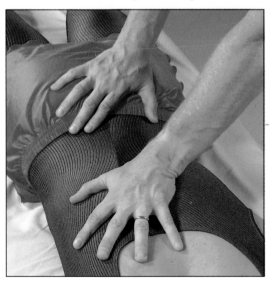

Apply compression with a twisting motion.

Take time to address the lower and upper back, hamstrings, and gluteals.

# *Muscle Broadening*

Muscle broadening is an effective but noninvasive way to spread muscle fibers, allowing freer movement.

Place the palms of your hands along and parallel to the muscle. Your thumbs should be an inch or two apart. Keep in mind that the muscle fibers generally run from joint to joint, so in order to spread the fibers, you should exert pressure across the muscle, not lengthwise.

While you maintain a direct compression by using your body weight, move your hands slowly away from one another. Make sure that you are engaging the underlying muscles and not just sliding over the skin. This action will spread the muscle fibers initiating a powerful circulatory response.

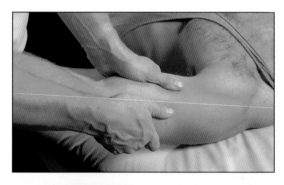

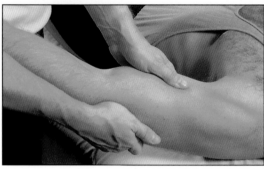

Apply compression to the muscle with the heels of your hands while keeping your thumbs parallel.

Repeat this technique so that the entire area of each limb is covered.

This technique is most suitable for spreading the muscle fibers of the arms and legs.

# Muscle Pumping

This powerful circulatory technique is great for decongesting tired muscles or for preparing an athlete prior to an event or workout. It generates a quick blood flow to the muscles—so it is also great for relief of muscle soreness after a heavy workout.

Deliver a rhythmic, pumping pressure to the musculature using the heel of one or both hands reinforced with the weight of your own body. As you compress the muscles, deoxygenated blood and toxins will be squeezed out. As you release the compression, freshly oxygenated blood and nutrients will rush in. Use rapid strokes for a stimulating Warm-Up Massage session and slower strokes for a Cool-Down Massage session.

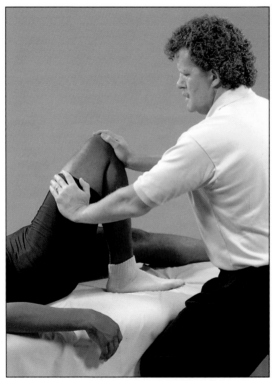

Use leverage to apply pressure.

Use this technique on the erectors (the muscles that run along the spine), hamstrings, tibialis anterior, and iliotibial band.

Take time to work slowly and thoroughly over the back. Spend additional time on tight or sore areas.

# *Direct Thumb Pressure*

Direct thumb pressure is an effective way to neutralize localized areas of spasm and tenderness. One of the major causes of muscle pain is interruption of blood flow caused by contracted muscles. The application of direct pressure will stimulate local circulation and can often dramatically relieve this type of pain.

Use one or both thumbs reinforced with the body's weight to apply direct pressure for 10 seconds. Sink in slowly so that the muscles have a chance to adapt to the pressure gradually. If you start out with maximum pressure, the recipient may tense to "guard" the area, and you will not achieve the desired effect of pain reduction.

Work well within the individual's pain threshold.

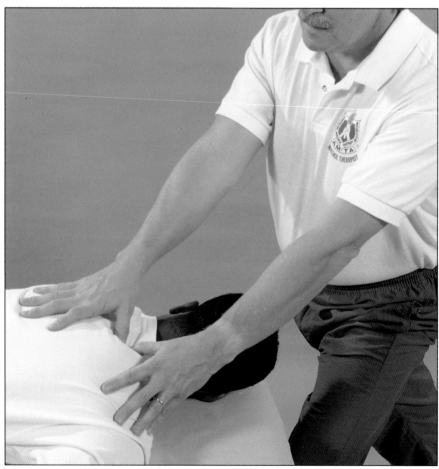

Use your leverage to apply pressure with your thumbs.

# Fist and Knuckle Twisting

Use the "high impact" technique of fist and knuckle twisting to unwind and loosen heavily layered muscles.

Use the flat area of your fist (the area between the knuckles and the first joint of the fingers) to engage the muscle tissue. Using your body's weight, sink into the tissue with a slight twisting motion that includes your wrist, arm, and shoulder.

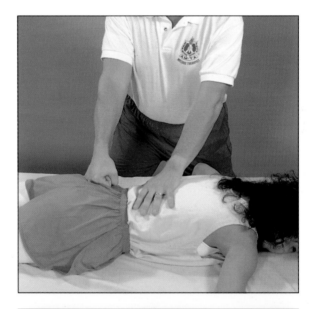

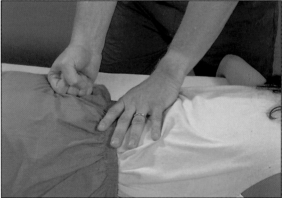

Use a loosely held fist to apply twisting compression.

This technique is especially effective on the gluteals and hamstrings.

## *Variation:  Bent Knuckle*

Deeper, more specific pressure can be delivered by performing the fist and knuckle twist technique with the bent knuckle of the middle finger used as a wedge to engage deeper tissues.

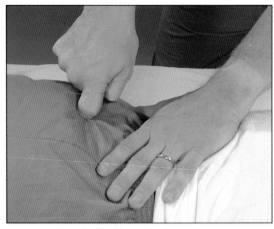

Use your knuckle to find tender points.

# Friction
## Broaden Muscle Fibers
## and Free Them From Adhesions

Friction techniques use the thumbs, fingertips, or palms of the hands to deliver firm pressure in a circular or back-and-forth motion in order to broaden specific muscle fibers and free them from adhesions.

# *Circular Friction*

Applying circular friction is a good way to loosen joints, tendons, and muscles.

The application of circular friction is a noninvasive way to work deeply into the muscles. To be effective, friction must penetrate through the skin and superficial fascia to the underlying musculature.

Place the fingertips of one hand on the body part you will be working on. (You can place the fingers of the other hand on top of your massaging hand to provide additional pressure and leverage.) Apply sufficient pressure so that your fingertips, reinforced by your body weight, sink through the skin and contact the muscle layer.

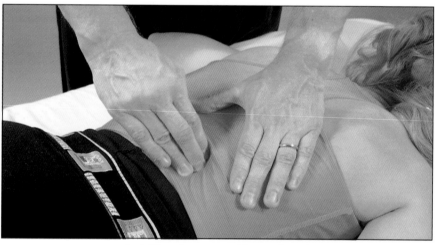

Stabilize the area with one hand
and perform 4-fingered circular friction with the other.

Maintaining this pressure, move your hand in quarter-sized circles, moving the skin along with it. Do not glide over the skin when you apply this technique.

Take time to work thoroughly over the musculature of the back, gluteals, and hamstrings. Do not work directly on the spinal bones, as this can cause discomfort.

## *Variation 1:   Splinted Finger*

For a more precise application, use a reinforced finger (middle finger placed on top of index finger) to apply circular friction to a small area.

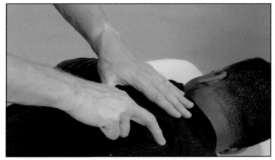

Place your middle finger over your index finger for precise application of pressure.

## *Variation 2:   Bent Knuckle*

For deep penetration, use the knuckle of your index finger to apply circular friction.

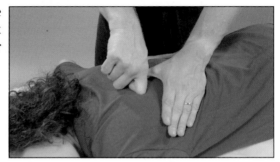

Use your knuckle for deeper penetration.

## *Variation 3:   Bear Claw*

To loosen a wide area, spread your fingers and thumb like claws to apply vibrating, circular friction.

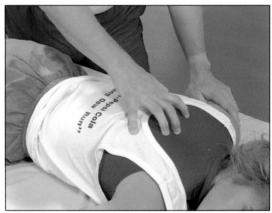

Spread your fingers and apply vibration to loosen the area.

# *Cross-Fiber Friction*

Apply cross-fiber friction directly on chronic soft-tissue injuries for pain relief and restoration of function.

Muscles subjected to overuse can suffer microtrauma that results in adhesions between the fibers. Adhesions restrict the natural broadening action of a muscle when it contracts, causing pain.

Deep fiber-spreading techniques manually separate individual muscle fibers and free the muscle from adhesions and scar tissue.

Standing at the side of the table, place your hands so that only the tips of your thumbs and fingers make contact with the body. Your palms should not touch the skin, and your thumbs should be positioned as pictured. Align your thumbs so that a back-and-forth sweep will be at a right angle to the muscle fibers you are working on.

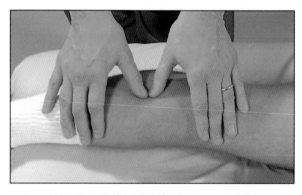

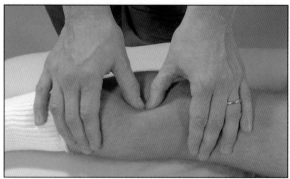

Use the tips of your thumb and fingers to sweep across the muscle at a right angle.

Cross-fiber friction can be readily applied to the erector spinae muscles, hamstrings, gastrocnemius, forearm muscles, and any areas commonly stressed by a particular activity.

## *Variation 1: Two Thumbs*

Use the tips of your thumbs to penetrate the tissues at a sufficient depth to engage the deeper muscle fibers. Sweep across the muscle fiber with a 1- to 2-inch stroke for up to 30 seconds, moving your thumb and hand as a unit. Movement should come from your hands and arms, not from your whole body. To be effective, cross-fiber friction must be applied at a right angle to muscle fibers and must be applied with sufficient pressure and penetration.

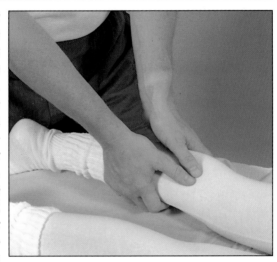

Use your thumbs
to engage deeper muscle fibers.

## *Variation 2: Four Fingers*

Use the fingertips of one or both hands, with your fingers held closely together, to apply a rhythmic, back-and-forth pressure at a right angle to the muscle fibers.

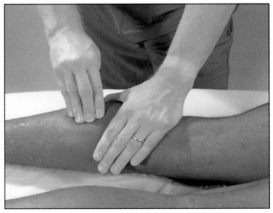

Apply back-and-forth pressure
with your fingertips.

## *Variation 3: Splinted Finger*

Place your middle finger over your index finger. Use the tips of the index fingers to apply a rhythmic, back-and-forth pressure at a right angle to the muscle fibers.

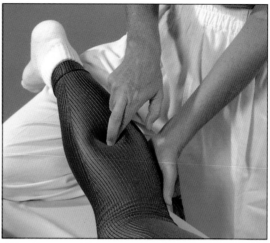

Reinforce your index finger by placing your middle finger above it, sweeping deeply across the muscle.

# Muscle Stretching
## Reduce Tension and Enhance Flexibility

Muscle stretching techniques are a unique aspect of Performance Massage. By combining these stretching movements with your hands-on techniques, you can initiate the following benefits:

- Reduce muscle tension.
- Initiate specific muscle relaxation and overall body awareness.
- Facilitate lengthening of tightened core, postural muscles.
- Enhance physical fitness by assisting joint flexibility.
- Reduce the risk of injury due to muscle imbalance.

When stretching any of your partner's limbs and joints, be sure to observe the following guidelines for maximum safety and effectiveness:

- Be sure the tissues have been warmed up before initiating your stretch.

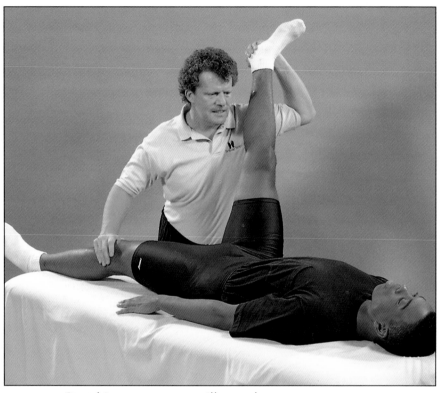

Stretching movements will complement your massage
if the tissues are warm.

- Use proper biomechanics and leverage, rather than arm strength, whenever lifting or stretching a limb. For example, if you want to stretch the hamstrings, stand at your partner's feet and lift his or her other leg, bending it at the hip. Rest the ankle on your shoulder, and place your right hand on top of the shin and your left hand just above the knee. Lean forward, keeping your partner's knee slightly bent, and stretch the leg toward the head. Move smoothly into the stretch, always respecting range of motion and muscle tightening. Hold the stretch for up to 20 seconds, and ask your partner to relax and breathe into the stretch.

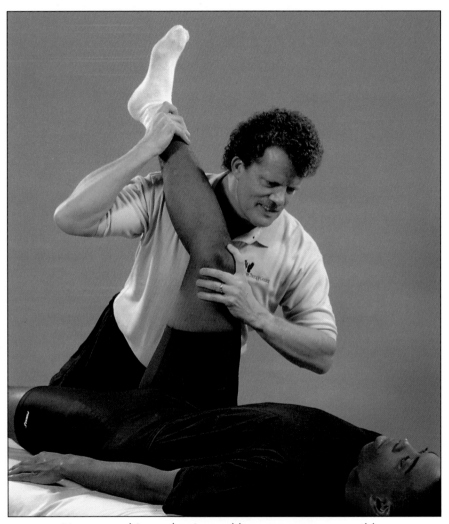

Use proper biomechanics and leverage, move smoothly, and hold the stretch while your partner relaxes and breathes.

- Stay in constant communication with the athlete.

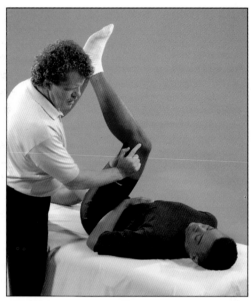

Communicate with your partner to ensure safe stretching.

- Ease in and out of stretches slowly and rhythmically.

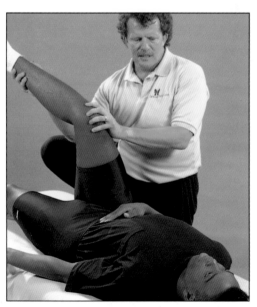

Move slowly and rhythmically to achieve a full stretch.

There are many specific muscle stretching techniques shown in the Performance Massage sequence that begins in chapter 6. The photographs and accompanying captions should be sufficient for you to learn them. Remember that a Performance Massage session should be intuitive and individualized to the recipient. You will probably invent additional muscle stretching techniques as you become more comfortable with giving a massage. Just be sure to follow the safe-stretching guidelines just listed.

## Chapter 6

# Head-To-Toe Massage Sequence

N ow that you are familiar with the essential techniques of Performance Massage, it is time to begin practicing the following sequence. By mastering this foundation, you will become skilled in a comprehensive full-body method uniquely designed to remove restrictions to free movement and optimal performance. As you become more experienced, you'll create sequences based on specific needs.

Study the illustrations as you practice these techniques, and respond to any feedback from your partner. Some abbreviated instructions are given to remind you of key points, but the page number where the techniques are taught in chapter 5 are also given in case you need to refer back.

This stage of learning is designed to produce an overall body massage of therapeutic potency. Practice each technique for three to five repetitions before moving on to the next stroke. This method allows you to develop a familiarity with each technique as you create a step-by-step total body approach.

# *Sequence*
## *for the Prone Position*

The following techniques are performed with the recipient in the prone, or face down, position. See page 48 for a description of how to position the recipient in the prone position.

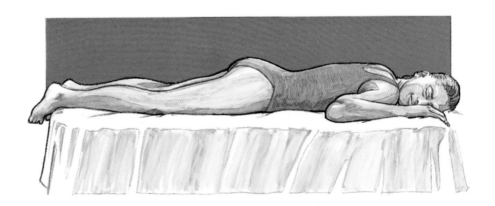

## Rocking (pages 56-57)

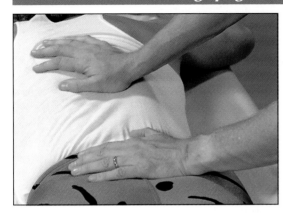

### Variation 1:
### Sacrum to low back

- Apply your hands to the natural contours of the sacrum and back.
- Initiate a gentle to-and-fro motion.

### Variation 2:
### Hamstrings to low back

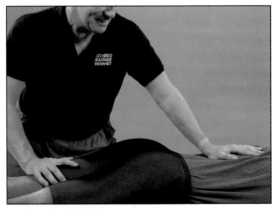

- Place the hands over the hamstrings and low back.
- Repeat the rocking motion.

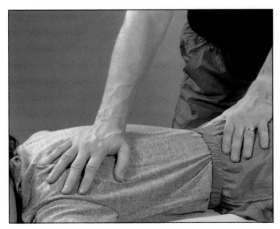

### Variation 3:
### Sacral stretching

- Apply steady pressure over the sacrum.
- Point your other hand upward.
- Create a stretch between the two points of contact.

## *Stretch and twist compression (page 71)*

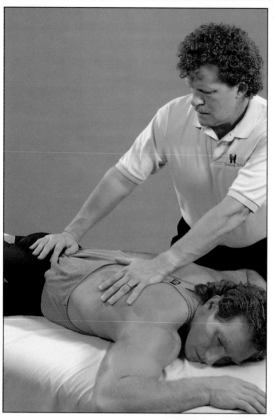

### Back

- Compress both hands into the back musculature.
- Initiate a gentle stretch in opposite directions.

### Sacrum

- Engage the sacrum with a firm holding pressure.
- Compress upward with your other hand.
- Twist gently in opposite directions

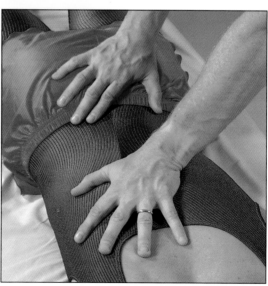

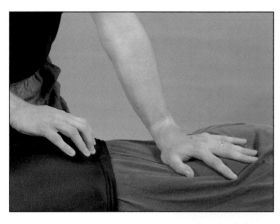

### Sacrum and back

- Curl your fingers onto the base of the sacrum and pull downward.
- Simultaneously apply upward compression throughout the back.

### Hamstrings and back

- Compress the hamstrings and the back simultaneously.
- Work both areas thoroughly.

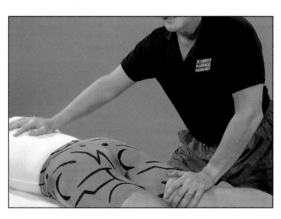

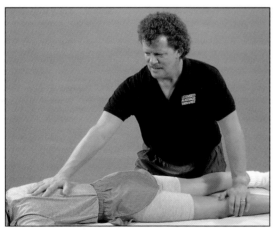

### Gastrocnemius and back

- Simultaneously compress the calf and mid-back region.
- Complete the twisting compression strokes with this maneuver.

## Skin rolling (page 64)

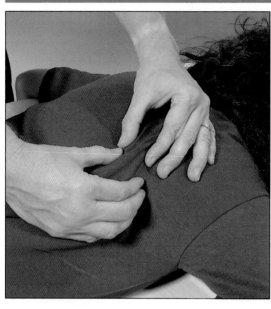

### Surface of back

- Twirl the clothing, skin, and superficial musculature between your thumbs and fingers of each hand.
- Cover the entire back.

## Fascial pickup (page 65)

### Lateral surface of back

- Grasp the superficial layer of skin and fascia.
- Gently pull upward.
- Wring the tissue between your thumb and fingers.

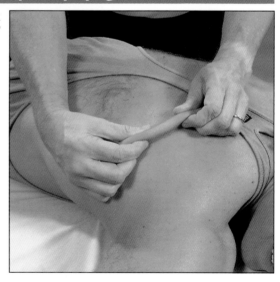

## Rotary thumb probe (pages 67-68)

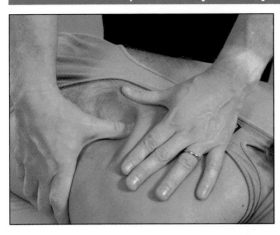

### Back

- Firmly compress the tissue with one hand.
- Sink the thumb of your other hand into the slackened tissue.
- Probe for areas of tenderness.

## Muscle broadening (page 72)

### Hamstrings

- Apply two-handed compression.
- Allow your hands to slowly spread apart.

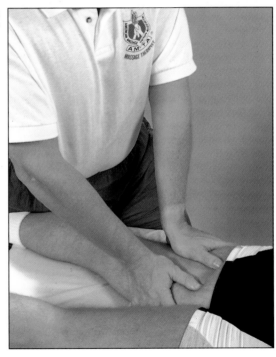

## Muscle pumping (page 73)

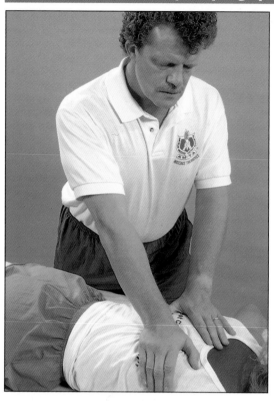

### Erectors

- Use the heel of your hand.
- Apply a series of rhythmic compressions over the paraspinal musculature.

## Kneading (page 63)

### Back of neck

- Knead the many layers of musculature at the back of the neck.
- Alternate grasping and releasing with each hand.

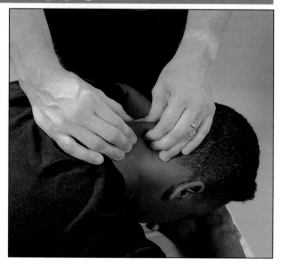

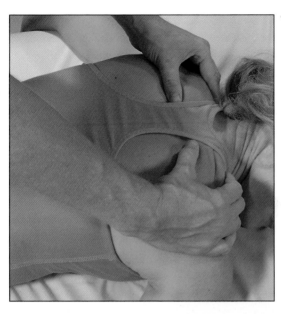

### Trapezius

- Roll and squeeze the musculature of the upper back.
- Use increasing pressure wherever you find tension, but stay well within your partner's pain threshold.

### Shoulders

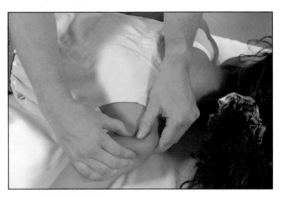

- Knead the deltoid muscles with both hands thoroughly.
- Work slowly in order to find areas of restriction and tenderness.

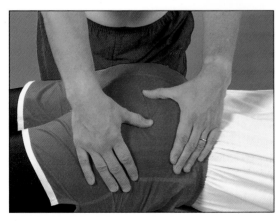

### Gluteals

- Assess for tenderness and tension.
- Knead the layers of gluteal musculature.
- Work thoroughly.

## *Pincer grip (page 66)*

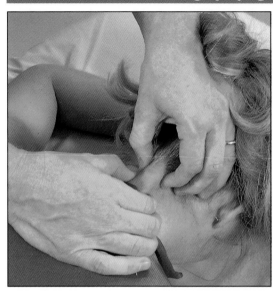

### Back of neck

- Compress into the neck musculature on both sides.
- Bring your fingertips and thumbs together.
- Hold with sustained pressure until the muscles release.

### Trapezius

- Perform a series of sustained squeezing movements over the trapezius.
- Hold until the layers of muscles begin to soften.

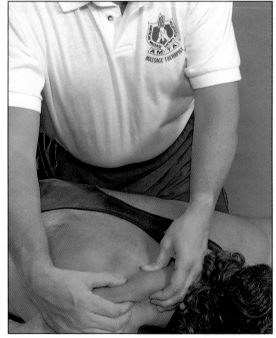

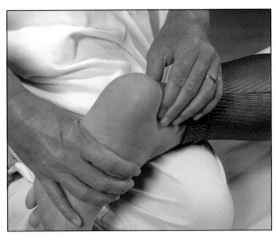

### Achilles tendon

- Apply a pincer squeeze to the Achilles tendon.
- Simultaneously stretch downward on the ankle.

## *Heel squeeze (page 69)*

### Hamstrings

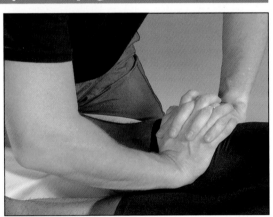

- Clasp both hands over the hamstrings.
- Bring the heels of your hands together.
- Squeeze and release in order to unknot tight muscles.

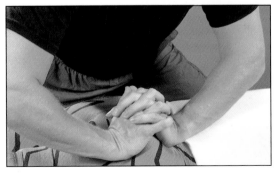

### Gluteals

- Perform a series of sustained heel squeeze movements to the gluteals.
- Be aware of releasing any tension and of hip tenderness.

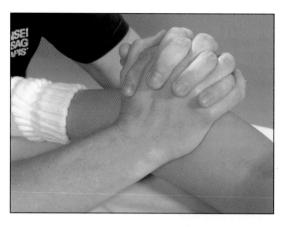

### Gastrocnemius

- Intertwine your fingers, bringing the heels of your hands together.
- Heel squeeze compression to the calf muscles is especially beneficial to runners

## Circular friction (pages 78-79)

### Variation 1: Splinted Finger
**Upper back**

- Perform circular pressure with your fingertips.
- Be aware of releasing painful knots in the upper back.

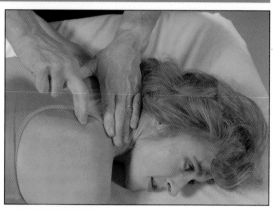

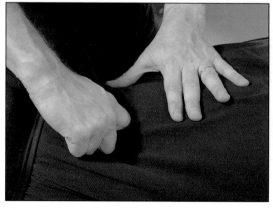

### Variation 2: Bent Knuckle
**Low back**

- Apply circular friction with your knuckles onto the lower back.
- Sink through the skin and contact the muscle layer.

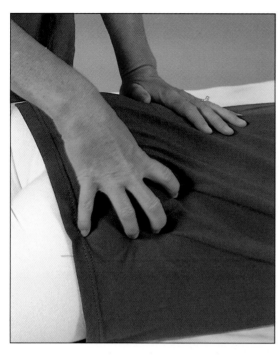

### *Variation 3: Bear Claw*
### Gluteals

- Spread your fingers and thumb like a bear claw.
- Apply vibrating, circular friction over the gluteals.
- Be aware of releasing deep muscle tension.

## *Fist and knuckle twisting (pages 75-76)*

### Gluteals

- Engage the gluteal muscles with a loosely held fist.
- Twist into the muscles, unwinding any constricted areas.

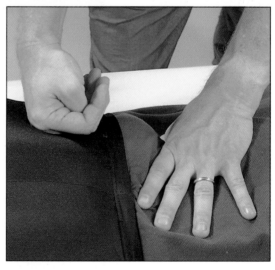

## *Cross-fiber friction (pages 80-82)*

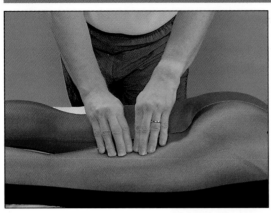

### *Variation 2: Four Fingers*
Hamstrings

- Use a rhythmic to-and-fro motion with your fingertips.
- Mechanically separate the fibers of the hamstrings.

### *Variation 2: Four Fingers*
Erectors

- Sink into the back musculature.
- Sweep back and forth over tight areas.
- Work slowly, assessing for tension.

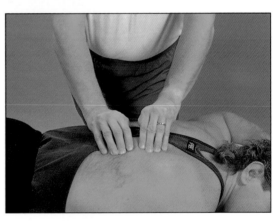

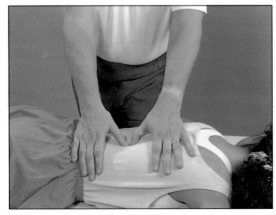

### *Variation 1: Two Thumbs*
Erectors

- Use both of your thumbs.
- Penetrate the tissues at a sufficient depth to engage deep muscle fibers.
- Be aware of knots and tension in the back musculature.

## *Direct thumb pressure (page 74)*

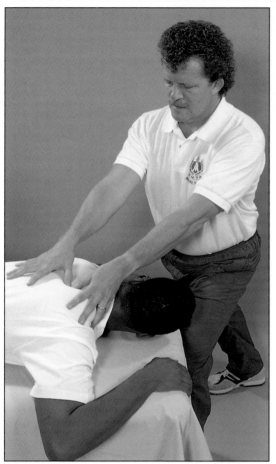

### Levator attachment

- Use both thumbs to isolate and compress trigger points in the upper back musculature.
- Hold for ten seconds.

### Rhomboids

- Sink your thumb into the rhomboid muscles, located between the spine and the scapula.
- Search for trigger points.

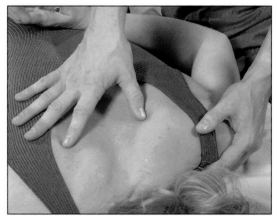

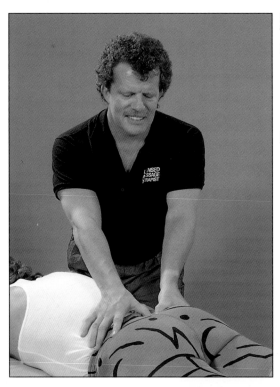

### Low back

- Apply firm holding pressure to trigger points or areas of tension in the low back.
- Hold for ten seconds to allow tenderness to subside.

### Hamstrings

- Apply direct thumb pressure to trigger points in the hamstrings.
- Keep good body mechanics as you lean into tender spots.

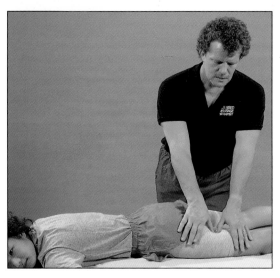

Perform the following muscle stretching techniques. Be sure to follow the guidelines on pages 84 to 86.

## Foot wedge

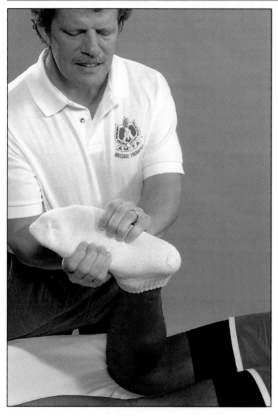

- Squeeze your finger-tips into the arches of the feet.
- Apply ten repetitions.
- Thoroughly address the soles of the feet.

## Ankle stretch

- Stabilize your partner's leg against your thigh.
- Move the ankle through its full range of motion.
- Include downward strokes at the ankle.

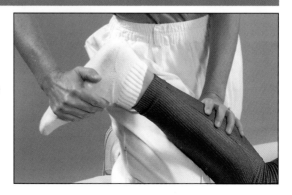

## *Quadriceps stretch*

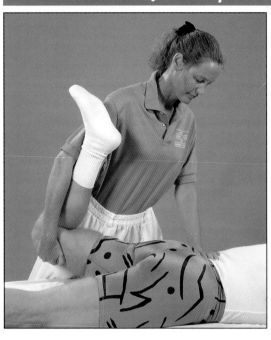

- Stabilize your partner's lower back.
- Flex your partner's knee and lift upward off the table.
- Perform five repetitions, gently increasing the stretch.

## *Hip scissors*

- Lift the hip upward and as you release it back to the table, perform twisting compression to the lower back musculature.

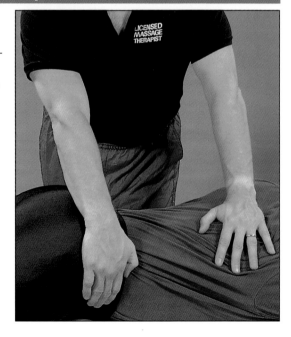

## *Shoulder release*

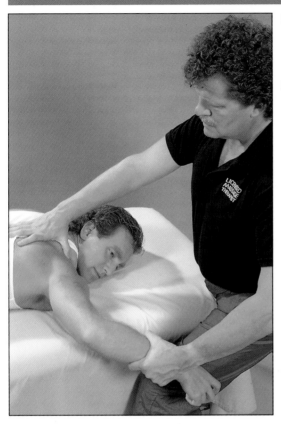

- Press the thumb of your table-side hand into trigger points in the upper back.
- Simultaneously stretch the arm and shoulder gently in circular motions with your other hand.

## *Opposite leg lift*

- Stabilize the lower back with palmar compression.
- Simultaneously lift your partner's leg (above the knee) off the table.

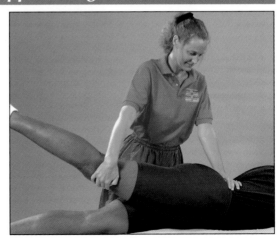

Conclude the sequence for the prone position with the following techniques.

## *Limb pull (page 58)*

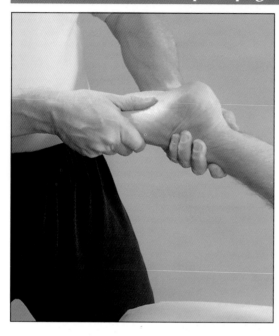

### Legs

- Stabilize the ankle.
- Grasp the foot.
- Exert a steady pull as you lean backward.

## *Shaking (pages 58-59)*

### Ankle

- Stabilize the foot with your thumbs in the arch.
- Simultaneously stretch the ankle with a slight vibration.

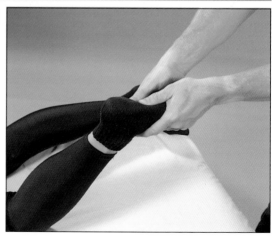

# Sequence
## *for the Side-Lying Position*

Now have your partner move into the side-lying position. See page 48 for a description of how to position your partner in the side-lying position. Bend one of your partner's legs, and perform these techniques.

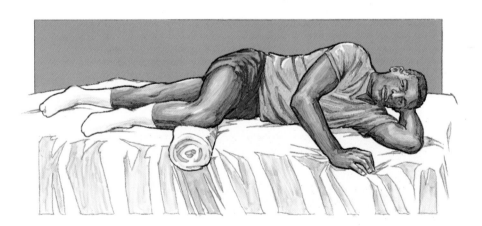

## Muscle broadening (page 72)

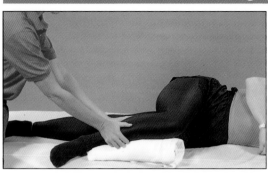

**Peroneals**

- Sink the heels of both hands into the lateral compartment of the leg.
- Slowly spread your hands apart to broaden the musculature.

## Fist and knuckle twisting (pages 75-76)

**Peroneals**

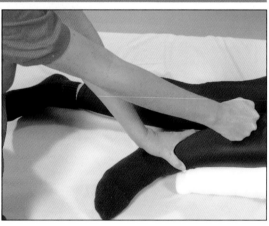

- Use a loosely held fist to release tightness in the musculature of the lower leg.
- Work with increasing pressure.
- Assess for areas of restriction.
- Gently twist into the tissue.

## Heel squeeze (page 69)

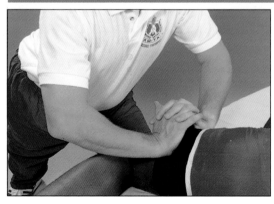

**Iliotibial band**

- Use both of your hands.
- Squeeze into the iliotibial band.
- Sustain pressure to reduce constriction and tension in this region.

## *Cross-fiber friction (pages 80-82)*

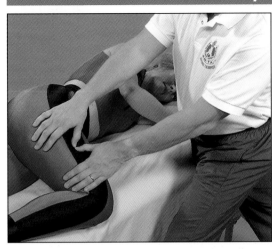

**Variation 1: Two Thumbs**
**Iliotibial band**

- Use your thumbs and both hands.
- Sweep back and forth until a softening occurs.

**Variation 2: Four Fingers**
**Iliotibial band**

- Use your fingertips.
- Sink into tightened bands of tissue.
- Sweep back and forth until a softening occurs.

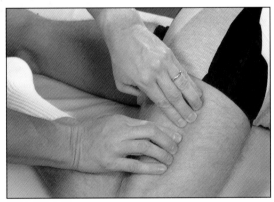

## *Fist and knuckle twisting (pages 75-76)*

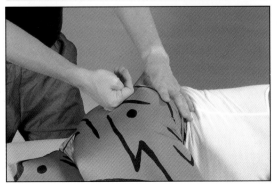

**Gluteals**

- Use the flat of your fist.
- Sink into the gluteal muscles with a slight twisting motion of your wrist, arm, and shoulder.

Perform these techniques on the straight leg:

## Muscle broadening (page 72)

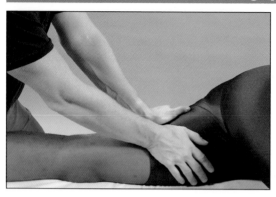

**Adductors**

- Sink into the adductor muscles of the inner thigh.
- Simultaneously slowly spread your hands apart.

## Muscle pumping (page 73)

**Adductors**

- Use the heel of your hand to muscle pump the adductors.
- Be aware of the increasing tissue release and pliability.

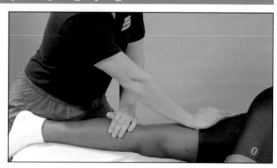

## Kneading (page 63)

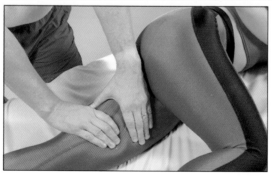

**Adductors**

- Perform kneading techniques on the inner thigh.
- Focus on any areas of soreness or tightness.

### Gastrocnemius

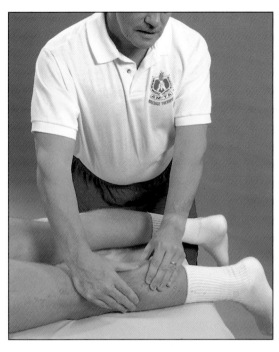

- Alternately squeeze and release the calf muscles.
- Work with increasing pressure to soften any restrictions.

Perform the following muscle stretching techniques, making sure to follow the safe-stretching guidelines on pages 84-86.

## *Hip extension*

- Stabilize the lower back.
- Simultaneously perform a slow extension stretch at the hip joint.

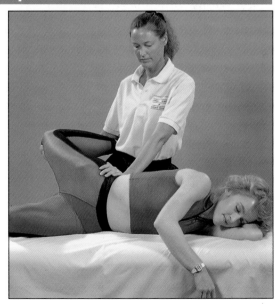

## *Gluteus medius stretch*

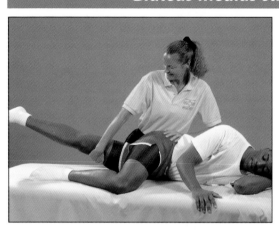

- Grasp your partner's extended leg above the knee.
- Lift your partner's extended leg off the table.
- Use your leverage to facilitate movement.

## *Torso twist*

- Gently compress the shoulder and hip joints in opposite directions.
- Take care to move slowly.

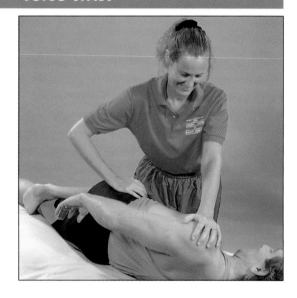

## Rib and shoulder stretch

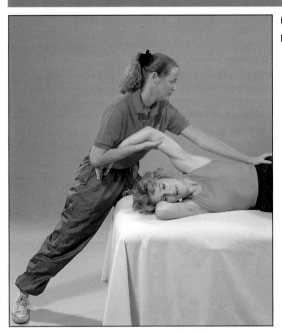

- Stabilize the hip.
- Simultaneously apply traction to the arm to decompress the thorax.

## Quadratus release

- Compress the extended leg off the table to the resistance barrier.
- Stabilize with your upper hand to further enhance stretching.

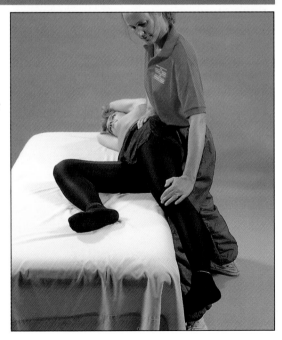

## *Scapula stretch*

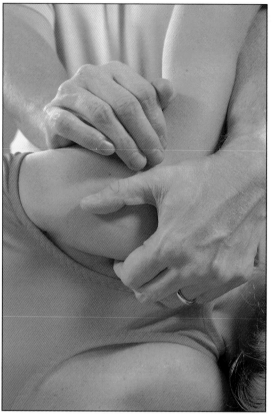

- Face your partner.
- Slowly retract the scapula.
- Allow fingertip compression along the attachments at the medial border.
- Be aware of adhesions and tender spots.

Now have your partner roll over to face the other direction. Bend the top leg and repeat the entire sequence.

# *Sequence*
## *for the Supine Position*

Now have your partner roll over into the supine, or face up, position, and proceed with the following techniques. See page 47 for a description of the supine position.

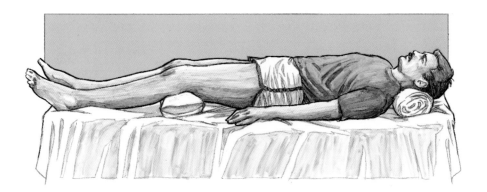

Begin the sequence for the supine position by working on the lower body.

## Limb pull with vibration (page 58)

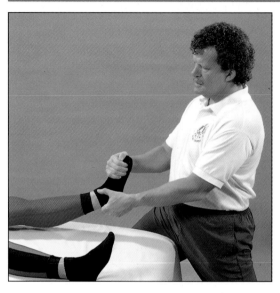

### Legs

- Hold the leg firmly and lean back.
- Use leverage and not arm strength.

## Rocking (pages 56-57)

### Legs

- Use the heel and fingertips of both hands.
- Rock both legs, applying a to-and-fro motion.

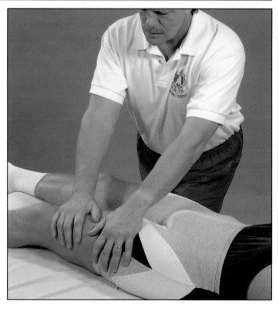

## Muscle pumping (page 73)

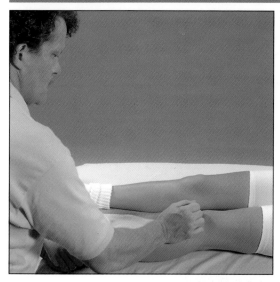

### Lower leg

- Compress alongside the tibia to enhance muscle softening.
- Be careful not to press on the bone.

## Fist and knuckle twisting (pages 75-76)

**Lower leg**

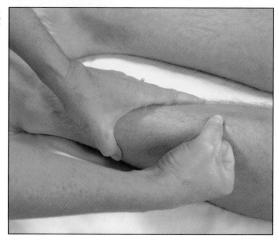

- Make a fist.
- Use the knuckles of one hand while stabilizing the leg with the other hand.
- Sink your knuckles with a twisting motion into areas of sensitivity or soreness.

## *Direct thumb pressure (page 74)*

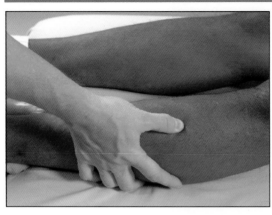

**Lower leg**

- Apply direct thumb pressure to trigger points for ten seconds.
- Work well within your partner's pain threshold.

## *Heel squeeze (page 69)*

### Foot

- Intertwine your fingers.
- Apply a squeezing compression to the foot.

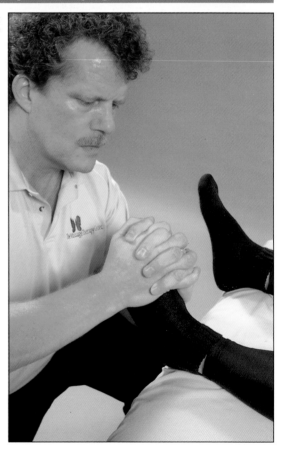

## *Fist and knuckle twisting (pages 75-76)*

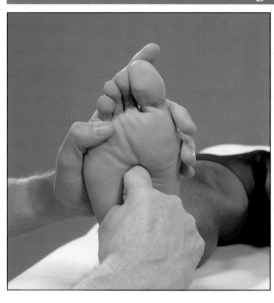

### Arch

- Stabilize the foot.
- Apply a twisting knuckle compression.
- Search for adhesions or areas of tissue density.

## *Direct thumb pressure (page 74)*

### Arch

- Apply the trigger point procedure with your thumb.
- Apply for ten seconds.
- Focus on dissipating tenderness.

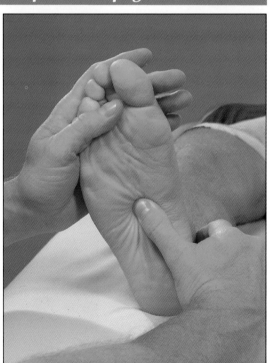

## *Muscle broadening (page 72)*

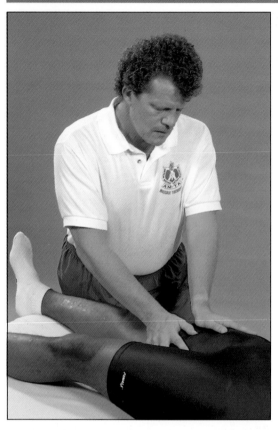

### Quadriceps

- Apply open-handed pressure.
- Slowly spread your hands apart.

## *Muscle pumping (page 73)*

### Outer quadriceps

- Use the heel of your hand.
- Compress the lateral quadricep muscle and the iliotibial band.
- Sink into areas of tissue density.
- Work from the hip to the knee.

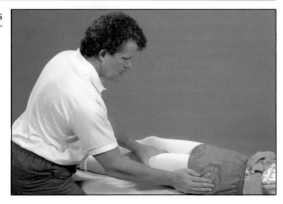

## *Kneading (page 63)*

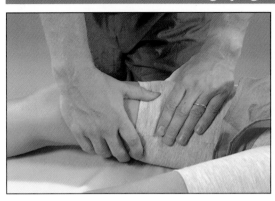

### Adductors

- Carefully squeeze and release the inner thigh musculature.
- Alternate hand movements.
- Decongest the tissue.

## *Cross-fiber friction (pages 80-82)*

*Variation 3: Splinted Finger*
**Around knee**

- Sweep your fingertips back and forth.
- Mechanically separate adhered tissues.

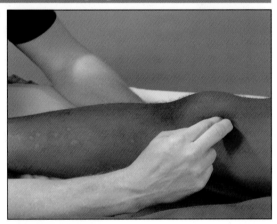

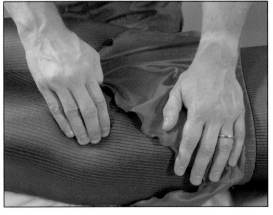

*Variation 2: Four Fingers*
**Quadriceps**

- Use your fingertips.
- Isolate any taut bands with high impact cross-fiber friction.

## *Direct thumb pressure (page 74)*

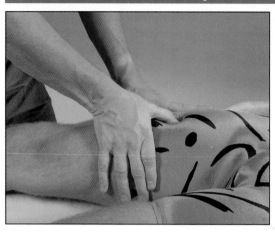

### Quadriceps

- Apply both thumbs directly into trigger points.
- Hold for ten seconds.
- Be sure to check adjacent tissues for additional tender spots.

## *Shaking (pages 58-59)*

### Leg

- Firmly grasp the leg.
- Lean back.
- Gently vibrate or shake your arms to initiate unwinding.

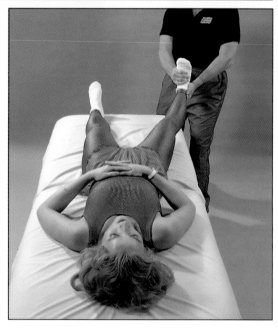

Continue the supine sequence by working on the upper body.

## *Limb pull (page 58)*

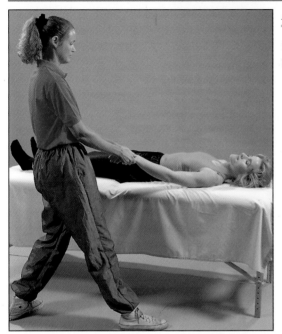

### Arm

- Firmly grasp the arm.
- Lean back using your leverage to decompress the musculature.

## *Heel squeeze (page 69)*

### Hands

- Intertwine your fingers.
- Apply a grasping squeeze to your partner's hands.

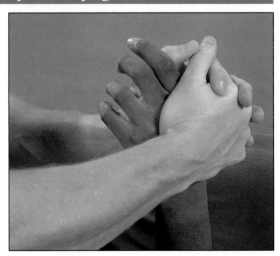

## Direct thumb pressure (page 74)

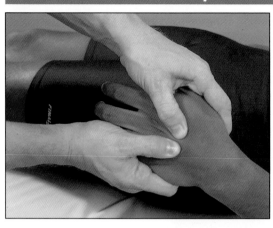

### Hands

- Isolate any areas of tension or soreness with your thumbs.
- Compress areas for ten seconds.

## Muscle pumping (page 73)

### Forearms

- Use the heel of your hand.
- Apply a series of compressions into the forearm musculature.

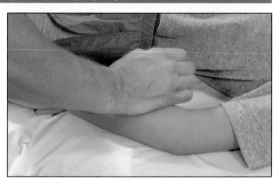

## Cross-fiber friction (pages 80-82)

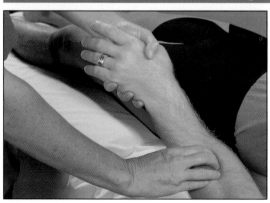

### Variation 2: Four Fingers
### Forearms

- Use your fingertips.
- Sweep across any tight bands within the muscles of the forearm.

## *Kneading (page 63)*

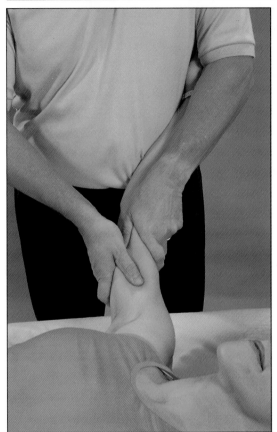

**Upper arm**

- Wring, roll, squeeze and release the muscles using both of your hands.
- Alternate hand movements.
- Decongest the tissue.

**Shoulder**

- Wring and squeeze the trapezius muscle of the upper back.
- Decongest the tissue.
- Spend additional time on areas of tension or soreness.

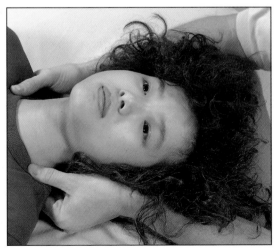

## Pincer grip (page 66)

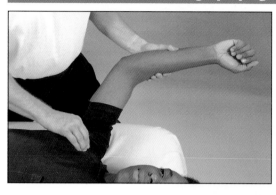

### Pectorals

- Gently grasp the lateral border of the pectoralis major.
- Place your thumb beneath and your fingertips atop the muscle.
- Slowly apply pressure while stretching the arm.

## Circular friction (pages 78-79)

***Variation 1: Splinted finger***
**Back of neck**

- Use the splinted-finger technique.
- Apply circular friction to tender spots on the back of the neck.

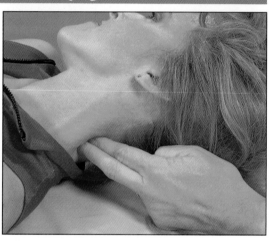

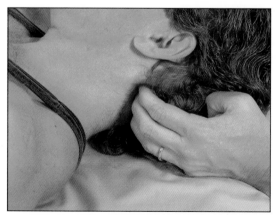

### Base of skull

- Use the basic circular friction technique with four fingers.
- Move your hand in quarter-sized circles at the base of the skull.
- Do not glide over the skin, but move the skin as you move your hand.

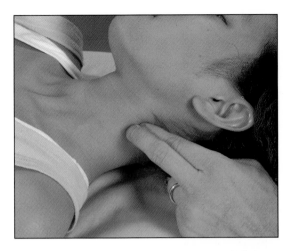

***Variation 1: Splinted Finger***
Side of neck

- Use the fingertips of your upturned hand.
- Work the small and often tense muscles at the side of the ` neck.

Masseter

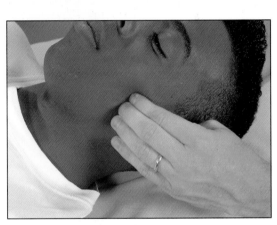

- Slowly wedge all four fingertips into the masseter muscle.
- Sweep in a circular motion assessing for tension.

## *Cross-fiber friction (pages 80-82)*

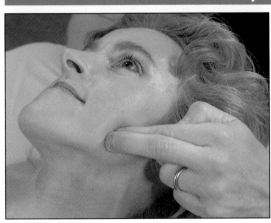

***Variation 3: Splinted Finger***
Masseter

- Use a splinted finger to identify taut bands within the masseter.
- Sweep across the fibers until the tissue softens.

## *Circular friction (pages 78-79)*

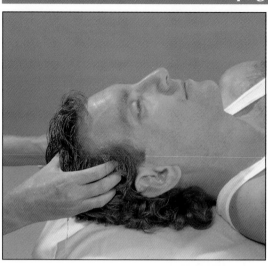

**Temporalis**

- Employ circular friction with your fingertips.
- Move the scalp over the skull.

Perform the following muscle stretching techniques. Remember to follow the guidelines on pages 84 to 86.

## *Masseter opening stretch*

- Curl your fingertips under the cheek bones.
- Your partner should slowly open and close his or her mouth while undergoing this maneuver.

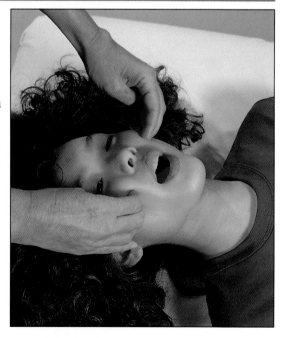

## Head and shoulder stretch

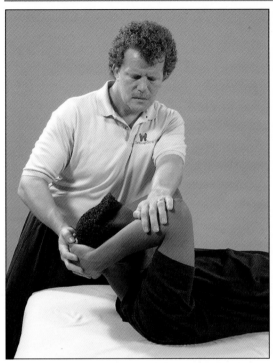

- Have your partner clasp his or her hands behind the head.
- Lift your partner's head off the table.
- Simultaneously add pressure to the elbows with your forearm.

## Neck flexion

- Slowly raise and lower your partner's head
from the table.
- Use a secure grip.

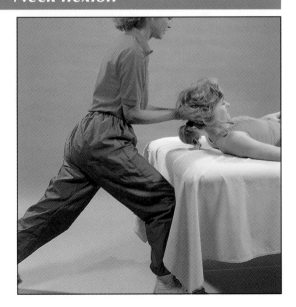

## *Ear to shoulder*

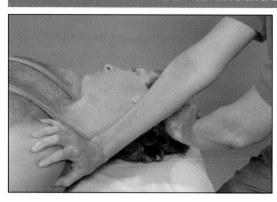

- Imagine a line running from your partner's ear to his or her shoulder.
- Elongate the line by gently but firmly pushing the head toward the opposite shoulder.
- This technique is an effective stretch for the neck.

## *Scapula release*

- Lift your partner's scapula off the table.
- Slide your other hand beneath the scapula.
- Curl your fingertips upward beneath your partner's scapula.
- Stretch the arm to the side.

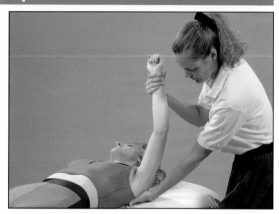

a

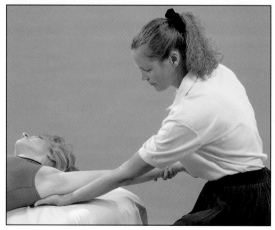

b

## Pectoral stretch

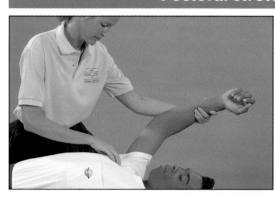

- Apply four-fingered pressure into the pectoral region.
- Simultaneously stretch the arm upward.

## Arm stretch

- Slowly pull your partner's arm across the chest.
- Stretch the outer region of the deltoid muscle.

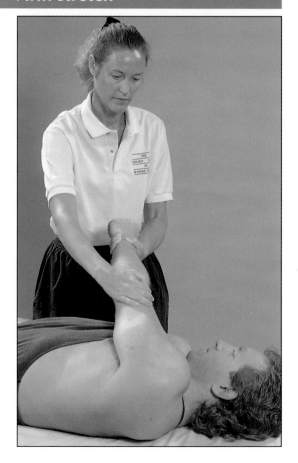

## Wrist twist

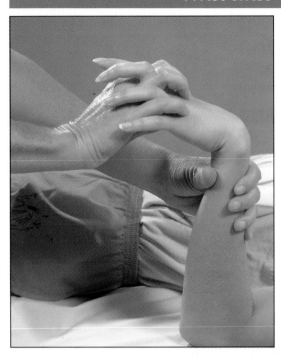

- Intertwine your fingers with your partner's.
- Stabilize your partner's wrist.
- Perform slow range of motion movements.

## Knee to chest

- Flex your partner's knee toward the chest.
- Move the knee to ward the other shoulder in a circular motion.
- Return to the starting position.

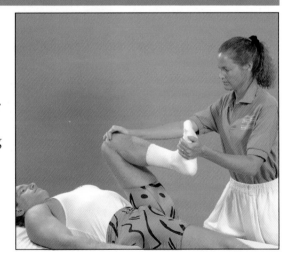

## *Gluteal stretch*

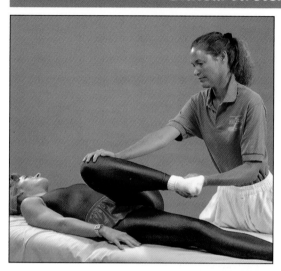

- Move your partner's flexed leg to the opposite shoulder or until a barrier is reached.
- Hold for up to thirty seconds.

## *Piriformis stretch*

- Point your partner's flexed knee to the opposite shoulder.
- Move the ankle away from you on an even plane with the knee.
- Hold for 30 seconds to maximize the stretch of the hip rotators.

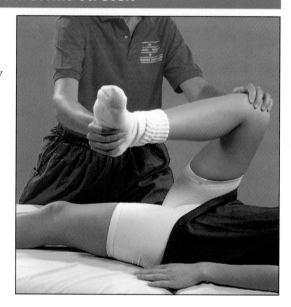

## *Adductor stretch*

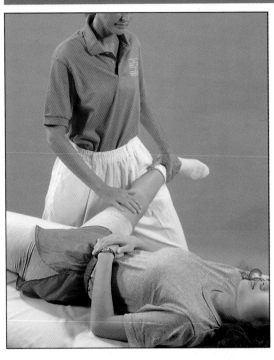

- Stabilize your partner's knee.
- Stretch away from the midline

## *Hamstrings stretch*

- Slightly bend your partner's knee.
- Lift the leg straight up until a physical barrier is reached.

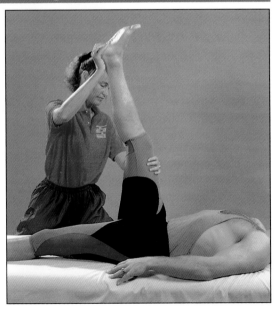

## Gastrocnemius stretch

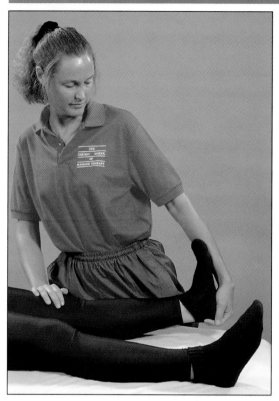

- Use a sustained grip.
- Flex your partner's foot upwards.

## Ankle stretch

- Stabilize your partner's ankle.
- Move the foot through a "figure 8" motion.

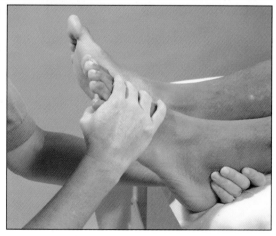

Conclude this Performance Massage sequence with the following techniques.

## Kneading (page 63)

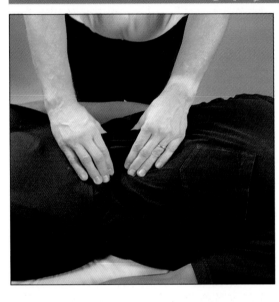

### Abdomen

- Perform rhythmical kneading movements over the abdomen to relax the abdominal musculature.
- Alternate hand movements.

## Abdominal sandwich (page 61)

- Sandwich the abdomen between your hands.
- Have your partner raise your upper hand by breathing deeply.

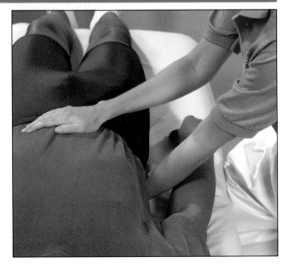

## *Stretch and twist compression (page 71)*

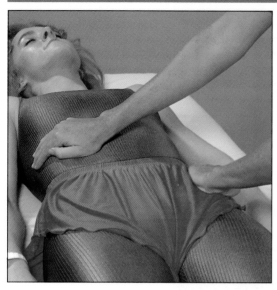

### Rib cage

- Gently compress over the natural contours of the rib cage and upper legs.
- Push your hands in opposite directions, assessing for areas of tenderness.

## *Shaking (pages 58-59)*

### Arms

- Grasp your partner's hand, keeping your thumbs on top.
- Keep your grip below the wrist.
- Lean slightly backward and shake the arm.

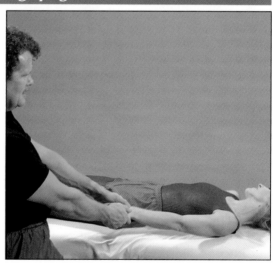

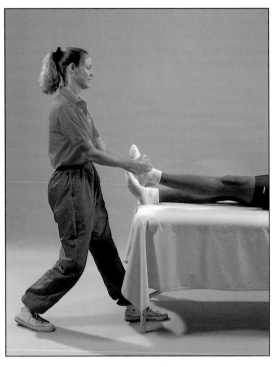

### Legs

- Grasp the foot and stabilize the heel.
- Lean back and gently shake your arms.

As you develop an understanding of and familiarity with the preceding techniques, try to perform at least 10 full-body sessions utilizing all of the strokes. You will find that this is hardly the 20-minute session we referred to earlier in the book. In all likelihood, the sequence will take an hour or more to perform. As you develop proficiency and begin to apply your efforts to individuals, you will find that your sessions will be more activity-specific; that is, you will concentrate your efforts on the areas susceptible to stress and breakdown characteristics of the activities the recipients engage in.

It is, however, a good idea to at least apply the basic compression and stretching movements to unaffected parts of the body in order to create a whole-body massage experience. The recipient will be less focused on areas of breakdown and will have an experience of being completely and thoroughly revitalized.

# *Appendix A*

# Resources

## Massage Table Manufacturing Companies

The three table manufacturers listed here provide not only state-of-the-art products but also written guarantees and excellent follow-up service. A massage table will probably be your biggest investment in your practice of Performance Massage. I strongly suggest that you purchase an adjustable and portable table in order to best develop your expertise.

For further information regarding bodywork tables and accessories or to find a dealer nearest you, contact Oakworks Inc., P.O. Box 99, 34 Main Street, Glen Rock, Pennsylvania 17327 (telephone: 717-235-6807); Touch America, Inc., P.O. Box 1304, Hillsborough, North Carolina 27278 (telephones: 1-800-678-6824 or 919-732-6116); or Blue Ridge Tables, Inc., P.O. Box 1833, 1123 S. John Street, Corinth, Mississippi 38834 (telephone: 1-800-447-2723).

# American Massage Therapy Association

Massage therapy is currently one of the fastest growing fields within health care. Being a professional massage therapist is a fulfilling and personally rewarding career that offers you a unique opportunity to positively influence the lives and well-being of your clients.

Contact the American Massage Therapy Association at 1130 West North Shore Avenue, Chicago, Illinois 60626 (telephone: 312-761-AMTA) for additional information regarding sports massage, a directory of AMTA-affiliated schools, and state chapter locations, or a free copy of "A Guide to Massage Therapy in America."

# Massage Publications:

The Bodywork Entrepreneur
  584 Castro Street #373
  San Francisco, CA 94114

Massage Magazine
  NOAH Publishing Co.
  PO Box 1500
  Davis, CA 95617

The Massage Therapy Journal
  AMTA
  1130 W. North Shore Ave.
  Chicago, IL 60626

The Maryland Bodywork Reporter
  13407 Tower Road
  Thurmont, MD 21788

# Anatomy Reference:

Elson, M. and Kapit, W. (1977). *The Anatomy Coloring Book*. New York: HarperCollins.

# General Massage Reading:

Beck, M. (1988). *Theory and Practice of Therapeutic Massage*. Tarrytown, NY: Milady Publishers.

Benjamin, B.E. (1978). *Are You Tense? The Benjamin System of Muscular Therapy*. New York: Pantheon.

Tappan, F.M. (1988). *Healing Massage Techniques*. 2nd. ed. East Norwalk, CT: Appleton and Lange.

# Anatomical Information

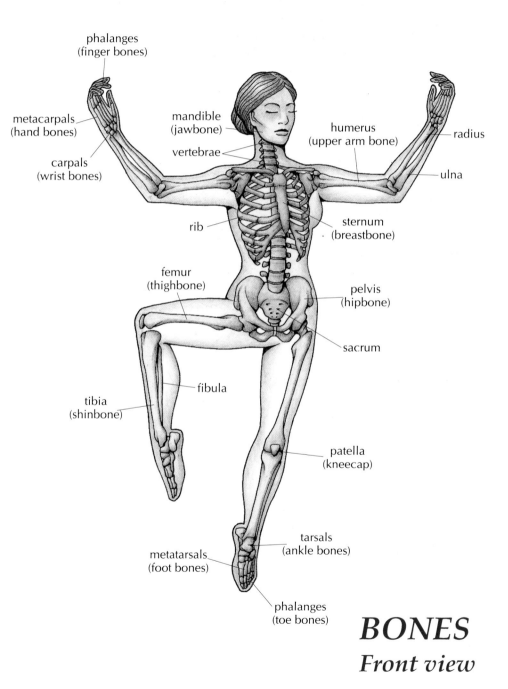

phalanges
(finger bones)

metacarpals
(hand bones)

carpals
(wrist bones)

mandible
(jawbone)

vertebrae

humerus
(upper arm bone)

radius

ulna

rib

sternum
(breastbone)

femur
(thighbone)

pelvis
(hipbone)

sacrum

fibula

tibia
(shinbone)

patella
(kneecap)

metatarsals
(foot bones)

tarsals
(ankle bones)

phalanges
(toe bones)

# BONES
*Front view*

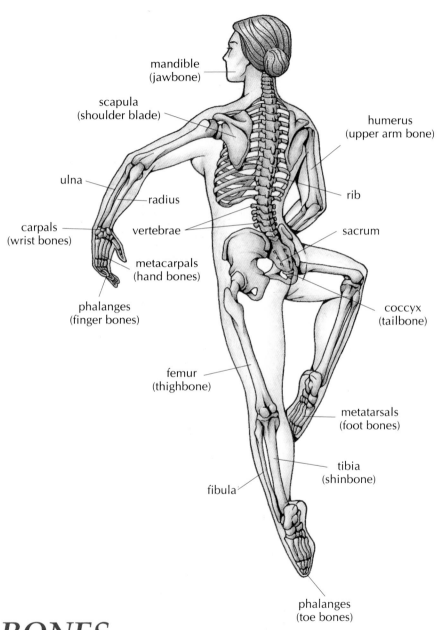

mandible
(jawbone)

scapula
(shoulder blade)

humerus
(upper arm bone)

ulna

radius

rib

carpals
(wrist bones)

vertebrae

sacrum

metacarpals
(hand bones)

phalanges
(finger bones)

coccyx
(tailbone)

femur
(thighbone)

metatarsals
(foot bones)

tibia
(shinbone)

fibula

phalanges
(toe bones)

# BONES
*Rear view*

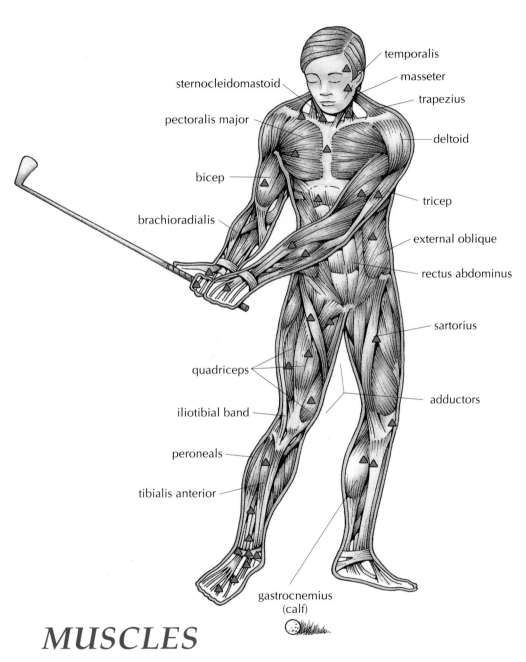

temporalis

masseter

trapezius

deltoid

sternocleidomastoid

pectoralis major

bicep

brachioradialis

tricep

external oblique

rectus abdominus

sartorius

quadriceps

adductors

iliotibial band

peroneals

tibialis anterior

gastrocnemius
(calf)

# MUSCLES
*Front view*

▲ = **trigger point**

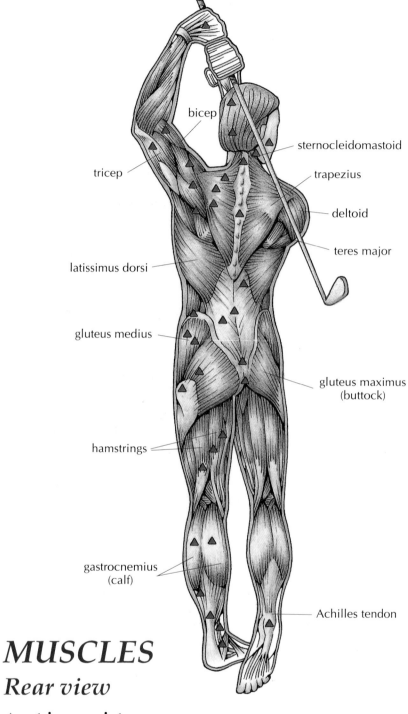

bicep

sternocleidomastoid

tricep

trapezius

deltoid

teres major

latissimus dorsi

gluteus medius

gluteus maximus
(buttock)

hamstrings

gastrocnemius
(calf)

Achilles tendon

# MUSCLES
## *Rear view*

▲ = **trigger point**

# Index

# *About the Author*

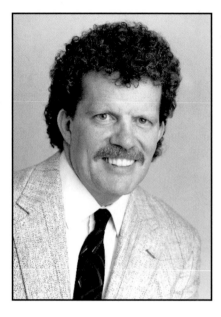

*A*s a former competitive weightlifter, boxer, and runner, Robert K. King has personally experienced the reality of coping with muscle strains and maintaining peak performance. For over 20 years he has worked as a professional massage therapist with many world class athletes, dancers, and entertainers such as Joan Benoit-Samuelson, Chuck Norris, and Mikhail Baryshnikov.

Mr. King is co-founder and director of the Chicago School of Massage Therapy, the largest state-approved vocational massage therapy school in the Midwest. Since 1977 he has held various offices in the American Massage Therapy Association (AMTA), including Illinois Chapter President, National Director of Education, and two terms as National President. He is also the co-founder and former National Examiner for the AMTA National Sports Massage Team.

As President of AMTA, King developed the AMTA Strategic Plan for Professional Development, resulting in increased public acceptance of massage therapy and a doubling in association membership.

As the former National Director of Education for AMTA, he spearheaded a national drive to help increase educational standards and upgrade school curriculums and continuing education programs.

Robert King is the author of several articles, essays, and instructional manuals including *Body Mobilization Techniques*, a training manual for massage therapists. He also conducts workshops, lectures extensively at schools and hospitals, and appears frequently in national media. He has also completed two instructional videos which are used in massage therapy schools throughout the United States.

A resident of Chicago, Illinois, Mr. King is married to Kathie Taylor King, who is a frequent assistant in his national workshops.